Therapeutic Storytelling

101 Healing Stories
for Children

Susan Perrow

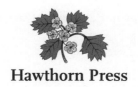

Hawthorn Press

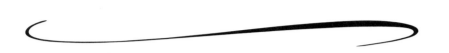

Published by Hawthorn Press, Hawthorn House,
1 Lansdown Lane, Stroud, Gloucestershire, GL5 1BJ, UK
www.hawthornpress.com

Therapeutic Storytelling © Hawthorn Press 2012
Cover photo © 'Rainbow over Africa' by Valerie A. de Vincent
Typesetting and cover design by Bookcraft Ltd, Stroud, Gloucestershire
Reprinted 2022 by Short Run Press Ltd, Exeter.

British Library Cataloguing in Publication Data applied for

ISBN 978-1-907359-15-6
eISBN: 978-1-907359-49-1

Contents

Dedication

For all children – everywhere …

Acknowledgements

Thank you to my children for their enduring love and encouragement of my 'story' passion.

Thanks to my kind, supportive and loving husband and a special thanks for his opportune work contract at Ololo Lodge in Kenya … providing me with the ultimate writer's retreat: a tent on the edge of a national park overlooking an acacia forest and a hillside of wildlife!

Thank you to Martin Large and Matthew Barton for their committed and thorough editorial work and their honest and encouraging feedback.

Thank you to fellow writer Annie Barratt for many helpful discussions on the challenges and joys of our lonely profession.

Thank you to my friend and colleague Sandra Frain for enthusiastic and inspirational conversations about stories and storytelling.

Thank you to the 22 teachers, parents and therapists who took the time to share their stories and story outcomes with me, then generously agreed to contribute their stories to this book.

Therapeutic Storytelling

Endorsements of Susan Perrow's work

Susan Perrow's message is beautiful and powerful in its simplicity. Tell children stories and they will listen to the wisdom these stories have to offer. What more gentle and effective way to reach 'our' children can we as parents and professionals ask for? This is essential learning for parents and all those who find themselves responsible for the care and development of children.
Christina Crawford, Educational Psychologist, Ireland

The therapeutic workshop was great! I got a lot of joy out of watching the beaming and smiling faces of the 90 attendees as they were leaving. They felt so empowered! The beauty of your ideas on Therapeutic Storytelling is that they are so simple to implement and *so amazingly effective*! Personally you have opened another door for me as far as the *imagination* of the child is concerned. Therapeutic storytelling will be another addition to our curriculum.
Bijal Shah, Principal of 'My School – Montessori', Nairobi, Kenya

Susan's therapeutic storytelling workshop gave life to the theory put forth in her book. Her stories are so beautifully written, so creative and soul touching. On the second day of the workshop many participants shared their stories specially written for their specific situation, it is a wonder that surprised the writers themselves since they have never thought they could do it. Through the workshop, Susan was so enthusiastic in sharing the wonderful results creative healing storytelling can bring, and helped us believe in our own capacity for story composing! With the book as a handbook that we can always refer to, life with our children will be more interesting and enjoyable!
Scarlet Cheng, Teacher/Parent, Beijing, China

The two workshops last weekend were *fantastic!* Thank you so much for a wonderful, entertaining, interesting, thought provoking and inspiring weekend. I think it went so well just because of who you are and your lovely open, non-judgemental and centred way of being. And of course because of the stories you told – just so engaging! I so love what you are doing with these stories – they are a rich tool to touch children's souls – what a blessing! I would love to be as fluent as you are in creating them. I am inspired to practice though.
Monique Rutherford , Child Psychotherapist & Parent Counsellor, Noosa, Queensland

The Therapeutic Storytelling workshop was very inspiring. Wide-ranging and helpful. This course may really make a difference to a lot of children's lives! Susan is an excellent teacher … clear, imaginative, uplifting.
Ursula Godber, Primary School Teacher, Ireland

Just a quick note to let you know how much I enjoyed your class on storytelling for children held here in Coffs Harbour. I was the only father there, which I felt was a waste, because as a father and a storyteller, I benefited greatly from your kind insights, advice and wisdom. Thanks for taking the time to help us be better parents.
Anthony Cougle, Parent, Moonee Beach, Australia

Though I often make up little stories and rhymes for my children, I have felt quite over-whelmed each time I wanted to come up with a story for a particular challenging behaviour or situation regarding my child. Your simple technique has taken the 'overwhelm' out of it and brought life and magic into writing a healing story. I look forward to my journey in therapeutic 'storying'. Thank you again for your 'healing' gift.

Shalini Christodoulou, Teacher/Parent, Singapore

I wanted to extend a deep thank you for sharing your gift and experiences – and acknowl-edge the inclusive way that you facilitated so that we could all find the storyteller within and all support each other. I feel like a juicy plum this morning – alive, inspired and positive – and also like I am on a very fertile, strong juicy plum tree sharing life's journey with so many other plums. I felt a oneness of universal consciousness in a way never before through your stories – the symbols and metaphors that we all connected with are so strong and timeless. Bless you and thank you.

Monique, Social Worker, Melbourne, Australia

Recently I was lucky enough to participate in one of Susan Perrow's therapeutic storytelling workshops held at our local school. Susan has a talent for both creating stories, and helping others to find their storytelling voice. She is a storyteller extraordinaire! Our day was envel-oped in 'metaphor'. I was instantly captivated! Susan shared many of her own personal stories and successes and a little of her journey, which held us all spellbound.

Susan took us through a process and story structure that helped us to write therapeutic stories and become a storyteller. Many people in the group were new to this idea, and to watch them leave with an extra boost of confidence and a spring in their step, as they put on their invisible storyteller hats, was just delightful. I know my hat received a big shiny polish!

Amber Greene, Educator, Writer and Parent, NSW, Australia

Word Angel

A poem from Africa written by Dr Claire Inala (Kenyan doctor and playwright – 'Healing with Words and Hands') after attending a Therapeutic Storytelling workshop

my friend the story teller
with her magic special gift
a treasured bless-ed healer
armed with words to mend the rift

between the heart & head & soul
that divides us all inside
she coaxes out our sacred dreams
(before you know it, you've complied)

and language is no barrier
to her rich enchanting spell
if you listen careful, closely
old, ancient wisdoms she will tell

she gathers hope and ties it up
in ribbons of coloured yarn
the telling of the woven tales
lifts e'en the most forlorn

a gentler salve could not be found
to ease the pain of life
Give Praises! for our precious one
mother, daughter, friend & wife.

Foreword

Therapeutic Storytelling

The 21st century is a time of great challenge and uncertainty. What can we offer our children and young people to prepare them for such uncertain futures?

The current pace of change is hard to keep up with, and we can easily feel we are living in a 'time pressure-cooker'. Since the Industrial Revolution, our concept of time – once grounded in natural cycles – has become dominated by economics, exemplified by such phrases as 'time is money,' or 'buying time'.

In our post-modern age, speed addiction comes to expression in fast foods, lightning-speed internet, instant global text messaging, speed-reading, and the 'three-quick-steps-to-spiritual-enlightenment' culture. To cope with all this there are drugs to help us keep up, and other drugs to calm us down again. As a psychologist, educator and futurist, I am only too aware of the short-termism that pervades our culture. As they rush their children from one activity to the next to ensure they remain 'competitive', I ask myself how much quality time do parents actually spend with them? An alarming number of parents today believe they 'don't have time to tell their children stories'. Affluent parents seem to have subscribed to the advertising myth that they can buy their children's happiness with the latest computer and mobile phone, and that ready-made screen images can replace imagination and the child's creative response to the world.

Yet what little children really need, more than anything, is to sit on their parents' lap, or on the floor at their feet, and listen to them telling stories. Susan Perrow knows this, and her book challenges us to realize it.

Children born in the last 10–15 years in affluent countries have never known a world without communication technologies of all kinds. Even in Africa, as Susan has found in her research there, television has replaced the grandmother in the role of family storyteller.

There is growing evidence that children who are overexposed to computers and other screen-mediated forms of communication become increasingly disconnected from the world around them. Paradoxically, all this 'connectivity' impedes real interaction with their human and natural surroundings. A growing number of kindergarten children have 'delayed' language, more than likely related to the reduction in face-to-face, and human-voice contact: an educational time bomb we can expect to see exploding over the coming decade.

Marshall McLuhan suggested decades ago that every advance in technology dulls a former human capacity. For example the increasing reliance of young people on email and mobile phone text messages for communication dramatically truncates the richness of living friendships. By contrast, a live storyteller sitting with children offers the rich nuances of voice, intonation, eye contact, gestures, facial expression, body language, emotional response and soul warmth.

Futurist and peace researcher Elise Boulding has suggested that the more vividly we can envision our preferred futures, the more likely we are to act to create that future. The more children's imaginations are stimulated through storytelling and the arts, the more they will develop the capacity to picture what they want for themselves and the world, and act creatively to achieve it.

Globally, regionally and locally there is a great need for new perspectives. Many people perceive current global tumults – environmental, psycho-social and political – as evidence of a breakdown of culture, and with it the loss of safety and comfort. Others, like myself, also perceive signs of a luminous breakthrough.

Susan Perrow's second book, *Therapeutic Storytelling*, is one of those signs of breakthrough that give us hope that we can actually transform some of the problems we have created for ourselves. Because of the fragmented and overly abstract style of education most of us have received, what we 'know' is often disconnected from our hearts, thwarting our courage and thus our ability to make creative changes. Susan shows us that stories can address this lack. Stories have the power to reconnect what we know in our heads with what we feel in our hearts; they can inspire, encourage and empower us to take the actions we know we must take to make this world a better place for future generations.

Stories can open and reconnect children with their hearts. This in itself is therapeutic. By addressing children's difficulties through their actual content, Susan's therapeutic stories go even further. This book will change the lives of children and at the same time inspire the adults who read it to create and tell more healing stories.

Jennifer M. Gidley PhD, Research Fellow, RMIT University, Melbourne. President of the World Futures Studies Federation

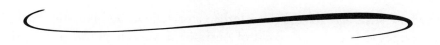

Introduction

Stories Know the Way

Many years ago an American Indian storyteller called Floating Eagle Feather visited the east coast of Australia. I was one of the privileged listeners at his storytelling session. He welcomed the audience by saying, *Some people think the world is made of atoms ... but I think the world is made of stories.*

I am still pondering this statement ... it was one of several catalysts that changed my life's path into that of a storyteller's quest. This quest, this path, this passion for storytelling, has wound its way through many levels and many stories – personal stories, family stories, community stories, my own writing, and stories from many cultures, past and present. Like the wellspring of stories for the world, it is infinite – I cannot begin to wonder where it will end. All I know is that my deepest satisfaction comes from connecting with others through stories.

In my first book of therapeutic stories, *Healing Stories for Challenging Behaviour,* I shared this passion through my experiences as a teacher and a parent, then I described a framework for writing therapeutic stories, followed by a collection of 80 stories for challenging behaviour and challenging situations. The book found its way into different parts of the world and has been translated into several languages. It opened new doors for me in my work and led (and is still leading!) me to run workshops in many different countries, from China to Africa, Europe to America, and across my own sunburnt land, Australia.

This second book, *Therapeutic Storytelling,* contains story ideas from these workshops (that I have developed into full stories), plus stories written by workshop participants (teachers, therapists and parents worldwide), plus some more stories from my own collection.

The aim of this book is twofold: to help you in the process of creating your own *healing* stories and to share with you many examples of completed stories that have the potential to address challenging situations and generally nurture and build character. The first section, Writing Therapeutic Stories, provides motivational thoughts and tips for creating your own stories to address challenging behaviour, offering a framework of 'metaphor, journey and resolution' and new ideas for therapeutic story writing … work in practice! The second section offers examples of the fruits of such work: 101 Therapeutic Stories for transforming a wide range of challenging behaviour and situations with children.

Categories for healing stories

The 101 stories are divided into different behaviour categories for easy reference – to work with directly, adapt, or use as models for the creation of your own tales. Each story is preceded by brief notes, including an age guide and suggestions for use. As in my first collection, the categories cover many forms of commonly identified challenging behaviour, from anger/aggression through dishonesty, obstinacy, and shyness/timidity to teasing and bullying. These categories also include some new themes identified in many workshops the world over, such as anxiety/insecurity, fussiness, intolerance, lack of confidence/resilience, silly/inappropriate speech, and difficulties relating to toileting/bedwetting.

Healing stories, not moralizing

In addressing what we regard as 'challenging behaviour' it is vital to enter imaginatively into the child's own experience rather than externally imposing a moral code in the form of 'cautionary tales' – i.e. working through fear of consequences. The *healing* approach gives the child an impetus to change forms of behaviour from within by developing imaginative metaphorical pictures that he makes his own – a much more durable and effective approach than merely urging conformity to external 'standards'. Healing stories stand at the very opposite end of the scale from the imposition of norms. They are gentle and child-friendly, respecting the child's own experience and affirming his desire and capacity to grow in all kinds of hidden and surprising ways.

There can never be a list of stories to suit every situation. 101 stories may sound like a comprehensive collection, but this is just the 'tip of the iceberg' of therapeutic stories. Behaviour is relational and contextual. It can rarely be addressed in isolation. Each child exists and develops within an intricate web of relationships and environments – family, school, community and global. It is you, the practising reader, who is in direct touch with the relationships, context and individual characteristics of the children whom you parent, counsel and teach; and therefore you alone are best placed to create stories for specific, individual needs. The first section, Writing Therapeutic Stories, is therefore intended to motivate you to become a story-maker yourself. The imaginative act of creating a story for a particular child or group communicates itself subtly to the children concerned. At some level they will feel affirmed by your care and effort.

In writing your own stories, a positive starting point is to hope that your healing story may simply help a situation ... and what a bonus if it can! I have learnt that the therapeutic story-maker should always work out of this 'helping' intention, with the occasional blessing that a story may indeed 'heal'. Even though this book is about 'healing' stories, I believe it is important to keep this 'helping' intention close to your writer's heart, and beware of an over-expectant or insistent attitude. There is unlikely to be any 'quick fix' for problem behaviour, and storytelling is just one of many possible therapeutic approaches and strategies.

Stories can't be seen as magic pills to heal or fix all problems. To thoroughly address the bigger picture requires a study of the complex 'tapestry' of discipline. Stories have the potential to be light-filled threads in this tapestry, but its underpinning threads are conscious and consistent approaches in caring for children.

Age range for stories

The 101 stories are mostly suitable for ages three through to ten years. It should be stressed however that stories don't have to be squeezed into a single age box. Sometimes a story written for a child may have a transformative effect on an adult. Sometimes an adult who is attending one of my workshops has an urgent need to write a story for their own adult situation, present and/or past. Examples of this are shared though the book. Ideas for using therapeutic stories with teenagers and adults are also included. My framework and techniques for writing stories can indeed be used for all ages.

Stories for global and community situations

As well as stories for challenging behaviour experienced at home and school, the range of examples in *Therapeutic Storytelling* include some for global, national and community challenges.

My work with therapeutic story-writing has led me to many countries over the years, and as I travel I encounter ever more requests for therapeutic stories specifically oriented to our 'global crises'. My first reaction to these requests was 'How can a story help here? World crises are too big for a story!' Then, after one fortnight in 2011, hearing of the horrendous earthquake in New Zealand followed by the tsunami in Japan, I felt motivated to give it a go! I was travelling in China at the time, without my trusty laptop, so I opened a real notebook, and picked up a real pen and started to write, following my framework of 'metaphor, journey and resolution'. Once my resolution was clear (*strength in caring, strength in togetherness*) the metaphors fell into place and *The Shadow Giant* was born (page 71).

Some stories for national situations include *The Rainbow Horses* (page 171), an anti-discrimination story written for the children of the new South Africa, and *The Rose and the Thorn* (page 74), a story for the children of Norway.

An example of community uses for stories is *The Sparkling River* (page 76). This was written after the devastation caused by the Brisbane River floods, to help give Brisbane children a sense of hope by understanding cycles of destruction and recovery. Another is *The Ants and the Storm* (page 75), a post-earthquake story for the children of Chengdu in China. Another is *The Keeper of the Lake* (page 239), written to encourage community involvement in the protection of a sacred aboriginal site near Byron Bay, Australia.

There seems to be no limit to where and how a story can help – anywhere and everywhere – stories know the way!

Stories know the way

In March 2011 I visited Beijing to run workshops and meet with the Chinese editor working on a translation of my first book. The Chinese version changed the title to *Stories Know the Way.* I was very happy to hear this. It captures the essence of my work with therapeutic story-making.

While in Beijing I was privileged to meet a Tao master and several Tao students who introduced me to an awareness of life and understanding that seems to correspond strongly with imaginative story-work. The Tao path creates conditions that favour 'letting things happen' (in a natural way) while many Westerners attempt to create conditions that 'make things happen'. This Tao path shows profound insight into a way of being that is humble, natural and simple.

The Tao intuition of 'the natural way' and 'natural simplicity' is a healthy foundation for story-making for children. Tao seems beyond words – I have been told it must be experienced first-hand to be known. However, in an attempt to capture it in language, the best description seems to be that it combines both feeling and thought. This resonates strongly with my personal experience of story-writing ... using my thoughts in a way that help me 'feel' a good story rather than intellectually plan it. This intuitive process is usually almost impossible to describe – I have only been able to suggest (to eager storytelling students) that once it has been experienced, it will be understood.

Walking in nature, being in nature, is usually the best way for me to 'feel' or 'hear' a new story. Mother Nature gives great help here – she offers a natural way into story-writing. The Bushmen people in Africa (my other home apart from Australia) also connect story with nature and feelings. They define a story as being ... *like the wind – it comes from a far-off place and we feel it.*[1]

Livo and Rietz, in their book *Storytelling: Process and Practice*, define a story as *an ancient, perhaps natural order of mind.*[2] This description seems to link directly with the Tao understanding of 'the natural way'. It certainly gives an insight into the importance of stories in our world, and the importance of our children hearing stories – in the past, present and future!

Stories feel the way, stories know the way, stories can find the way. Stories can find their way right into your soul, just as water finds a way through a crack in the wall when nothing else can! And like water, stories rejuvenate and are vital for healthy growth and development.

Many stories together make a 'well' for life travellers to dip into and continue on their journey, enlivened and refreshed ...

    ... travellers from Australia ... .
    ... travellers from Africa ... ...
    ... travellers from China ... .
    ... travellers from the East and travellers from the West ...
    ... travellers from the North and travellers from the South ...

I hope that the travellers who read this book will be enlivened and refreshed as they dip into the well of stories; and that these stories will find their way into them as a living, creative resource – one never fixed but ever-flowing. I also hope they will be encouraged to create their own 'stories that know the way'.

Susan Perrow
www.susanperrow.com

Section A
Writing Therapeutic Stories

1

A Construction Model for Story Writing

The aim of this section is to share a construction model for story-making that has helped me and many workshop participants create healing stories for children. This was outlined in my previous book but is presented here again with updated observations and experiences based on 'work in progress' over the last five years.

My intention is to provide a guide for story-making, but not a 'fail-safe formula' – stories are alive and don't like to be boxed or categorized. Time and time again with my story writing and in my workshops I find I make and then break any formulas or rules!

If there is any fixed guide at all, it is one that encourages 'intuit and play'. This requires letting go and playing – something that our often over-critical adult consciousness finds hard to do. The story-maker needs openness, trust and stillness of mind, 'letting things happen' (in a natural way) rather than trying too hard to 'make things happen'. As a story-maker I try to 'feel' a good story rather than plan it intellectually.

While very hard to describe such an intuitive process – as difficult perhaps as describing water – the first chapter in this section is a humble attempt to give the process some loose form and help readers to experience it.

The second chapter in this section, 'Getting the Story Juices Flowing', provides some ideas and exercises to help open up your creativity, and to encourage a playful approach to story-making.

Both chapters in this first section use my previous book as a foundation guide – there is detail to be found in *Healing Stories for Challenging Behaviour* that I have not repeated here – as in the chapters on 'Understanding Story and Behaviour', 'Different Stories for Different Ages', 'Truth and Morality' and a full section (five chapters) on 'The Art of Storytelling'. I recommend using this earlier book in conjunction with *Therapeutic Storytelling*.

What is a therapeutic story?

All stories are potentially healing or therapeutic. If a story makes people laugh or cry – or both! – the laughter and tears can be healing. Folk- and fairytales, through their universal themes and resolutions, have healing possibilities. They can offer hope and courage for facing the trials of life, affirming our capacity to change and develop.

David Suzuki, a world-renowned environmentalist, suggests that stories can help in 'healing' our earth by building a spiritual connection to 'place'. If a simple nature story, for example, can help connect children to their local beach, river or forest, they can become more conscious of protecting these and caring for them as they get older. Stories can help develop and strengthen our holistic relationship to the environment.

The very experience of listening to a story, no matter what the content, can be 'healing'. Regular storytelling sessions can develop and strengthen children's concentration, and activate their imaginations. These effects are a healing balm today when children frequently spend many hours in passive mode, watching TV and DVDs. A story requires and stimulates the imaginative creation of inner images, whereas the above media present a fixed, pre-created image that must be accepted by the viewer without invoking his own creative capacities.

Alongside this generally healing potential of stories, specific stories can help or heal behaviour in specific situations. For the purposes of this book, such stories are here described as 'therapeutic'.

If our definition of healing is to *restore to health, bring back into balance, become sound or whole,* then therapeutic stories can be described as *stories that help return balance and wholeness to a behaviour or situation that is out of balance.*

Therapeutic storytelling is a gentle, easy yet often very effective means of addressing difficult topics with children. The story form offers a healing medium that allows children to embark on an imaginative journey, rather than being lectured or directly addressed about their behaviour. By identifying with the main character or characters, the child is empowered as obstacles are overcome and a resolution achieved.

Stories are like natural or homeopathic remedies – and like natural medicine, they draw on the child's own latent forces and capacities to redress an imbalance. Sometimes, likewise, acceptance of storytelling is akin to the struggle for acceptance of natural medicines: common sense tells us that it should be welcomed with open arms, but the commercial and scientific world sets up huge opposition to this. Likewise, a more materialistic mindset finds it difficult to appreciate that a problem can be better dealt with by enlisting imponderable, hidden forces of the imagination than by tackling it head-on.

Fortunately this is slowly changing. From time immemorial story-telling has been used as a powerful educational and *healing* tool, and there is an exciting trend to re-awaken this age-old art form. A small but growing group of educational thinkers, researchers, teachers and practitioners now give due acknowledgement to expressive, imagina-tive ways of thinking and knowing, thus helping to revive the art of storytelling and use it in therapeutic ways.

My hope and vision is to once again have teachers and parents working with the power of story and the imagination in their role as mentors and guides to the children in their community, supporting the capacity of children through the medium they love and respond to best – the imagination. This capacity is, after all, what binds whole communities together and makes worthwhile human relationships possible, for it enables us to feel our way into others' experiences.

Weaving the framework

My construction model for writing a therapeutic (healing) story works with a three-part framework of 'metaphor', 'journey' and 'resolution'. It is helpful to identify and discuss these separately, even though they weave together intricately to create the finished story.

The framework put forward here is only one suggested approach. Some of the stories included in this book have not been written based on this (or any other) foundation but have followed their own intui-tive path … so please do not see it as the only way to write stories. It is offered as a starting point for story-making. It may also help you with de-constructing existing stories, and thus eventually feed into creating new stories. I encourage you to do this deconstruction exercise on some of your favourite folk- and fairytales – it may give greater clarity about their inner construction and composition.

Firstly you need to be clear what you are trying to achieve when writing a therapeutic story. A story devised to heal challenging behaviour does not involve making 'bad' behaviour 'good', or making 'naughty' children into 'good' ones. Instead it is about trying to recreate wholeness or balance in the child's own experience. It is also important to understand that children's behaviour, like all human behaviour, is contextual and relational. Any particular behaviour can rarely be effectively addressed in isolation (see *Healing Stories for Challenging Behaviour* for an in-depth chapter on 'Understanding Behaviour'). When working with children's challenging behaviour, storytelling is just one of many possible approaches and strategies – one thread in the whole fabric.

When writing a healing story it helps to carefully select therapeutic metaphors and to construct a journey or quest to meet the need of the situation *and* the age of the child or children. The story should very definitely not have the aim of moralizing or inducing guilt – this cannot be stressed enough! The objective is to simply reflect what is happening and, through the story 'metaphors' and 'journey', offer ways to work with and very slowly change the behaviour, and provide a realistic resolution. If the process is too goal-oriented it not only becomes over-intellectual but at the same time less effective. Behaviour often lives deeply in us as habit, and this can only change by allowing insights and imaginative pictures to sink down into the depths of the will and, unseen there, work their mysteriously transformative effects.

A healing tale should, as much as possible, leave the listener free to come to her or his own conclusion – in this way the 'power of story' is left to work its own magic. As Ben Okri suggests, leave the story to do its work 'in silence, invisibly':

> *It is easy to forget how mysterious and mighty stories are. They do their work in silence, invisibly. They work with all the internal materials of the mind and self. They become part of you while changing you.*[3]

Positive resolutions

The resolution in a therapeutic story is the restoration of harmony or balance in a situation or behaviour that has been disruptive or out of balance. Even though the resolution comes at the end of the story, when planning it is usually helpful to think about this before anything else. If the resolution is not clear, then it is difficult to know what to work towards with your metaphors and journey. Hence my decision to discuss this aspect of the framework first!

It is important for a resolution to offer affirmation rather than inducing guilt. For example, in the story of *The Elephant's Trunk* (page 67), the hitting behaviour is out of balance and unacceptable to Tembo's brothers and sisters. They try to stay clear of him as he bashes and thrashes his way through the day. They can't trust what he might do with his strong trunk. Then Tembo falls down slippery rocks. His bashing and thrashing can't help him here and he finds himself stuck in a pool at the bottom of the cliffs, far below his family. With the help of Old Grandmother Elephant and the 'rope' made from elephants' trunks and tails, Tembo is finally rescued. The story, with the use of both obstacle and helping metaphors (discussed on page 67), offers a simple transformational journey from 'using one's strength to hurt' to 'using one's strength to help'. The little elephant is not made to feel guilty about his behaviour. Instead the story journey leads naturally to a positive resolution in which balance and harmony are restored. By contrast, Rudyard Kipling's otherwise delightful story about the elephant's trunk in *Just So Stories* only redresses the balance at the end by giving power to hurt to the little elephant who was previously on the receiving end of it, and therefore cannot be seen as a therapeutic story in the true sense.

In the story of *Little Wolf,* (page 158), the mother's efforts (to encourage the young wolf to join in with the rest of the pack and learn the ways of the wolf clan) come to nothing. Yet the young wolf's lack of interest in everything is clearly out of balance. Can you imagine a wolf just sitting down in the snow, paws over his ears, eyes squeezed shut? By undergoing the journey of capture in the hunter's trap, the out-of-balance experience is taken to an extreme and then resolved when the wolf is rescued and set free to run with the rest of the wolf pack. What a relief for Little Wolf and what a relief for the listener!

Different kinds of behaviour and different situations seem to require different approaches. Some are quite straightforward – for example, in a story for a child who is continually using swear-words or 'bad language', the obvious resolution is to have the swearing replaced by more constructive uses of 'voice'. In *The Singing Snake and the Dancing Bear* (page 212), the snake ends up using his voice to sing beautiful songs.

A more complex approach is presented in the story of *The Rainbow Horses*, an anti-discrimination story written for the children of the new South Africa (page 171). The story leads the listener through conflicts of intolerance and pride. Slowly the tiny grey clouds created by the conflicts cover the sky, the rain begins, and the land is flooded. A common need for shelter brings the horses together in a cave high in the mountains. Finally they give up their rainbow-coloured manes to help weave wings for the golden horse so it can fly across the sky and bring back the sunshine. The transformative resolution here is through intolerant behaviour changing to 'accepting' or tolerant behaviour by individual choice, rather than external punishment or enforcement.

A less obvious resolution occurs in a story for a child with separated parents. This needs some careful thought – the story shouldn't offer more hope than real life – i.e. don't suggest that the parents come back together! To help plan the resolution, some questioning may be necessary. Do the parents communicate and share time with the child? Has one parent disappeared altogether from the family scene? There could also be a chance for the parents themselves to hear a message in the story and change their behaviour – perhaps learning about consistency and the need to keep the child's needs to the fore. Perhaps the story could be about a mother and a father fish living in two different rock pools or two different lagoons. The child could move from one pool to the other through a seaweed and coral pathway. Perhaps the seaweed whispers a special song? A parent could use this song while driving the child to spend time with the other parent. This could help to minimize the anxiety that often arises at such 'hand-over' times. The story could also include the metaphor of the strong sunlight being filtered through the water and giving light to each rock pool at different times. If it is not suitable for the two rock pools to be close (perhaps the parents are a long distance from each other, physically and/or emotionally), they could be on opposite sides of a wide reef, or there could be some rocky headlands and beaches (or a wide stretch of ocean!) between one and the other. Working out these different journeys and resolutions can be a healing balm for the parents and the therapist/teacher, as well as for the child.

For a story to help a child with a friend or family member who is terminally ill (or who has already died), it would be inappropriate to make up stories where the sick get better and live happily ever after. The story-maker has a serious responsibility to try to capture the bigger picture, with the resolution taking the listener to a place higher than, or different from the earthly one. Parents writing for their own children would most likely work from their own religious and/or philosophical beliefs. Teachers or therapists writing a story need to take the family's beliefs into account. See the stories *The Butterfly* (page 101), *Grandfather's Cloak of Light* (page 100), *The Rainbow Dove* (page 104) and *The Oriole and the Cherry Tree* (page 99) for four different examples.

No matter how simple or complex the story journey, it is essential that the ending or resolution be happy and hope-filled. Good triumphing over evil is a very profound theme in folk- and fairytales, and likewise in therapeutic stories, and children the world over need to hear this hope-filled message. Only slowly should we introduce the genre of 'real' stories with unhappy endings. Older children, in late primary school or high school, who are studying the lives of famous people, are ready to meet the harsh reality of early explorers suffering gruelling deaths by starvation, or war stories full of desolation and despair. Older children can cope with sad or tragic endings. But in making your choices, don't forget that older children, and teenagers, and adults too, also need the satisfaction and nourishment of a 'happy ending' from time to time. In therapeutic work, especially, they need it more often than not!

Examples of positive resolutions

Story	Out of balance behaviour/situation	Resolution – back into balance
The Shadow Giant (page 71)	Greed and power is dominant	Strength in caring, strength in togetherness
The Ants and the Storm (page 75)	Children anxious following an earthquake that collapsed their kindergarten building and some homes	Reassurance that teachers and parents will protect them
The Rhythm Sticks (page 50)	Continual loud behaviour	Control of noise; polarity and rhythms with noise
The Not-So-Perfect House (page 85)	Overly perfect; anxious if things are not perfect	More relaxed; understands that things can't always be perfect and this is okay
The Wombat Family (page 112)	Three-and-a-half-year-old still wanting to drink mother's milk; mother exhausted and not wanting this any more; mother also wanting child to bond more with father	Child loses interest in suckling; child becomes more independent and enjoys having new adventures with his dad
The Ocean Playground (page 117)	Clumsy and chaotic play	More careful and constructive play

Story	Out of balance behaviour/situation	Resolution – back into balance
A Family of Snails (page 142)	Anxious about leaving the family home	Content with two homes; excited about the journey back and forth from one to another
The Gnomes and the Golden Crowns (page 181)	Fearful, lacking in confidence and resilience	Strength and courage
Little Wolf (page 158)	Always complaining, never happy about anything	Becomes interested and motivated
The Boy and the Pearly White Shell (page 216)	Inability to listen; non-stop talking	Learns to listen
The Shy Robot (page 206)	Withdrawn, lack of confidence with speech	Becomes confident with speech
The Barnacle-Covered Fish (page 222)	Soiling pants; not using the toilet	Confident in using the toilet; experiences a new freedom
Clever Chameleon (page 88)	Continually teased; always a victim	Overcomes bullying; gains self-confidence
The Bowing Tree (page 115)	Greedy; lacking care for others	The joy of caring and sharing
The Winged Horse (page 177)	Insecure, unmotivated	Gains confidence and motivation
The Rainbow Horses (page 171)	Intolerance of differences	Acceptance of differences
The Digger that Always Says 'No'! (page 233)	Child 'stuck' in always saying 'no'	Child becomes 'unstuck', becomes more compliant and co-operative

The mystery and magic of metaphor

In simple terms, a metaphor shows us one thing as another, and in doing so extends the way we see the world, also often refreshing and enlivening our perception.

Using the medium of picture imagery, metaphor speaks directly to our imaginative faculties, bypassing our rational brain. Such metaphoric byways and pathways enable us to explore the ideas, forces and powers that lie behind or beyond our rational thought. Overcoming the limitations of our fixed categories and often cumbersome or clumsy everyday human language, metaphor, in a mysterious and magical process, offers a form of 'higher' or more holistic cognition:

> *Metaphor juxtaposes familiar concepts to reveal higher, archetypal concepts. These higher concepts cannot be literally stated in familiar language. The higher concepts are 'unnamed', no single definable word attaches to these 'thought beings' nor are they accessible to abstract, logical reasoning. They are poetical intuitions that incarnate into thought and language through the skilled manipulation of familiar concepts.[4]*

Metaphor is very different from simile. While simile compares one thing with another and highlights its resemblance using the word 'like' ('Your eyes are like stars'), metaphor accomplishes the magical transformation of turning something into something else ('Your eyes *are* stars'). In simile, the process of comparison involves our more rational brain, our thinking processes; whereas metaphor reaches deep into our psychic imagination and, simply stated, 'touches our heart'. In fact we can see this in child development. For a young child, living in imaginative worlds, an ordinary object such as a stick *becomes* a sword, a snake, a bridge, a wand or almost anything else (and sometimes all of these through the sequence of a game). When, in growing older, he starts to say that something is *like* something else, by contrast, he has emerged from the heartfelt immediacy of metaphorical unity to a more distanced point of view.

In *The Little Prince* we learn a simple secret from the fox:

> *And now here is my secret, a very simple secret:*
> *It is only with the heart that one can see rightly;*
> *What is essential is invisible to the eye.[5]*

Metaphor touches the heart and *it is only with the heart that one can see rightly.* For this reason metaphor has long been the language of mystics, spiritual teachers, poets, storytellers and other expressive art forms.

Let's explore one example of 'metaphor' – the *garden*. A quick glance through spiritual writings and poetry across the continents and throughout history shows that 'garden' metaphors are well-nigh limitless. Yet this is only one image drawn from a limitless source of metaphors!

Spiritual leaders and mystics continually use garden metaphors in their teachings. Sri Anandamayi Ma, a Bengali guru, writes about *One vast garden spread out all over the universe. All plants, all human beings, all higher mind bodies exist in this garden in various ways.*[6] Kahlil Gibran, the famous Lebanese poet, states that *Life without love is like a tree without blossoms or fruit.*[7] And in the Bible we read *Either make the tree good, and his fruit good; or else make the tree corrupt, and his fruit corrupt: for the tree is known by his fruit.*[8]

Many poets connect the garden with love and beauty, and in this context the image of the rose often stands supreme. In writing of my love for my own mother, I wrote a poem about *The rose in the garden of my life* that *Filled our days with her flower song … Her bloom, sweet and strong, To God's own treasure box belonged.* The metaphor of the rose in the garden captured everything I could possibly want to express about my love for my mother and the beauty of her devoted mothering.

However, there is more than lofty spiritualism, love and beauty to be found in 'garden' metaphors. Kipling, in his poem 'The Glory of the Garden', does not dwell on flowers and beauty, but uncovers the work behind this and finds *the tool- and potting-sheds … are the heart of all.* He writes that *such gardens are not made, by singing: 'Oh, how beautiful!' and sitting in the shade,* and that *half a proper gardener's work is done upon his knees.*

William Blake strikes yet another note in 'The Garden of Love'. Here he presents images of usurpation and lost paradise: not of sweet flowers, but of a chapel built on the green where he used to play … with *graves, and tombstones where flowers should be; and priests in black gowns … walking their rounds … binding with briars my joys and desires.*

The above examples illustrate – though very briefly and fleet-ingly – what an important and varied role metaphor has played in expressive human culture and communication. Metaphor speaks directly to the imagination, building its connections through feeling rather than theory or abstract reasoning. Integrated into storytelling, a metaphor, or many metaphors, can, as in spiritual writings and poetry, take on a mystery and magic, sometimes subtle, sometimes powerful. The metaphors often come alive and gain energy from each other in a vibrant and exciting interplay. Depending on the story journey, the same metaphors can assume different roles. For example, in one context a 'lagoon' can be an obstacle for a trapped whale to overcome; in another it can play a safe and helping role for a boat that has come to shelter from the storm. This of course reflects the fluid nature of life and the dynamic changes of meaning that occur depending on context and situation.

Obstacle and helping metaphors

As a vital ingredient in therapeutic story-making, metaphors help form imaginative connections that draw in and 'enchant' the listener. An integral part of the story journey, they often play both negative roles (obstacles, hindrances and tempters/temptations that help to pull a behaviour or situation out of balance) and positive roles (helpers or guides that bring the behaviour/situation back towards wholeness or balance). The following table of 'Metaphors in story-making' gives some examples of these (page 15), but firstly it may help to work through a few possible approaches.

Example one

Imagine a story written for a child who is using 'foul' language, which speaks directly of the problem: a child who is always swearing at others but learns to stop when other children refuse to be her/his friend. If told in class, because the story lacks metaphors to help 'lift' the listeners into their imagination, the teacher could be inter-rupted by someone calling out, 'Joshua does the same, he swears all the time!' It is even questionable whether such an example, devoid of metaphoric imagery, could be called a story.

Let us now take the same example and build a story with meta-phor. Starting first with 'simile' can be a helpful inroad into story-making. A swearing child could be compared, say, to a snake with a poisonous tongue. Then we drop the comparison ('as if', 'like'), creating metaphor instead, and use it to dive into the story: *There was once a beautiful snake that lived in a large and comfortable basket and travelled with the best circus in the land. This snake was a singing snake ...* (*The Singing Snake and the Dancing Bear*, page 212).

Now some of the 'obstacle' and 'helping' metaphors enter the story – the snake gets lazy with his performance and the crowds (an obstacle metaphor) begin to shout foul words back at him. The snake begins to copy them and finds that this gets him attention, even if in a negative way. But this behaviour is not fitting for a family circus, and the ringmaster calls on the wise dancing bear (a helping metaphor) to come up with a solution. The next metaphor along the story journey (another obstacle) is the grass weaving that forms a new lid for the top of the snake's basket. This creates a dark space inside and the snake falls into a deep sleep. When he wakes up he has to work hard to squeeze himself through the thick grass lid to get back out into the daylight, and on the way he loses his old skin, his old self. The resolution is the snake's 'self-progress' towards gaining a new coat, a new persona. The old skin has gone, and with his new and dazzling skin the snake now enjoys being a singing and dancing snake, joining in with the wise bear in a new act in the circus.

This story journey, with the use of obstacle and helping metaphors, shows the transformation from using one's voice in a negative way to using it in a positive way.

Example two

A story is required for a five-year-old boy who is continually hurting others with his hands. Having observed that one of this boy's favourite animals is the elephant, let us find our way into the story-making by starting with a simile: *A hitting hand is like the whacking of a wild elephant's trunk.*

Now we have a starting point we can dive right in. *There was once a young elephant called Tembo. Tembo was one of the strongest young elephants in the herd. But Tembo was always using his strong trunk to bash and thrash things* (*The Elephant's Trunk*, page 67).

Knowing that a five-year-old child loves rhyme and repetition, we use a rhythmic motif to accentuate the behaviour, and repeat it several times through our story: *Bash and thrash, bash and thrash, my trunk is so strong – I can bash and thrash.*

The bashing elephant's trunk (strengthened by rhythm and rhyme) is an 'obstacle' or 'hindrance' metaphor. The story journey takes us to a waterfall at the top of steep rocky cliffs (another obstacle). The elephant is trying to 'bash and thrash' his brother as he crosses the waterfall, and he falls down the slippery rocks into the pool below.

Enter, as 'a helping metaphor', Old Grandmother Elephant, who has tried to give guidance to Tembo before now – but Tembo did not want to listen. Now he is stuck in a pool of water at the bottom of the cliffs and is in dire need of assistance. The next 'helping' metaphor along the story journey is the rescue rope made from trunks and tails. This 'rope' formed by the combined strength of grandmother and Tembo's brothers successfully pulls Tembo to safety.

The story, with the use of both obstacle and helping metaphors, offers a simple transformational journey from 'using one's strength to hurt' to 'using one's strength to help'. Through a light and humorous approach, the story leads to a positive resolution and the behaviour is restored to balance.

More examples of metaphors in story-making

The table below lists examples of metaphors used in some of the therapeutic stories in this book. It is a guide only – the imaginative qualities of metaphor make them difficult to sort and categorise. You will notice that in one example, *A Family of Snails*, one of the 'obstacles' is also one of the 'helpers': it is an obstacle for the snail to leave the 'snug flowerpot' but by the end of the story it becomes one of the helping metaphors as the little snail realizes that he now has two homes – a snug flowerpot and a snug hole in the brick wall.

Metaphors can play different roles in different stories depending on the story context. Mother wombat's pouch in one kind of story could be a 'helping metaphor' but in the story of *The Wombat Family* it is a definite hindrance to baby wombat's development, and also a hindrance to the mother's relationship with her son; an octopus's tentacles could be a helping metaphor in a story where many hands were needed to make something, but in the story of *The Ocean Playground* the tentacles are presented as a clumsy obstacle (a metaphor for the child who kept knocking things down while playing).

In some stories, metaphors play quite definite and conscious roles, while in others they are more subtle. In *The Shadow Giant*, the owl, along with many other birds, sets out on a helping quest for the Queen of the Heavens; in *The Rainbow Horses* the golden horse drives away the grey clouds so the sun can shine upon the land once again. The owl and the golden horse play 'conscious' helping roles in these two stories. On the other hand, in *The Digger that Always Says 'No'*, the helping metaphor is quite unconscious – the children playing in the sandpit innocently show the digger 'how to be a digger'. This is not a conscious helping role on behalf of the boy and the girl, but it is enough to get the digger out of his stuck position and into movement (very similar to when a child is stuck in always saying 'no'!)

As an exercise in experiencing and understanding the use of metaphor in story-making, I suggest you read some folk- and fairytales, and some other stories from this book, then make up a table of your own, identifying both obstacles and the helpers.

But be forewarned! You may find a story that has metaphors that don't fit either of these categories. An interesting discovery at a recent workshop was that some metaphors seem to play a 'transitional' or 'transformational' role. For example, in the story of *The Singing Snake and the Dancing Bear*, the snake falls into a deep sleep inside his dark basket – this dark space and the metaphoric sleep play a transitional role in the story. In *The Digger that Always Says 'No'* the farmer stops for a cup of tea – this is a transition metaphor that gives time for a solution to present itself (and it does!). In the story of *The Boy and the Pearly White Shell*, the metaphor of 'sinking deep down to the bottom of the sea' offers a dark yet peaceful transformation for the loud behaviour of the boy.

I encourage you to explore this further – for me it is still work in process!

Metaphors in story-making

Story	Obstacles, hindrances, tempters	Helpers, guides
The Shadow Giant (page 71)	Destruction on the earth, in the ocean, in the air; large rock cavern; Giant's chant: *Greed is my game and Power is my name.*	Queen of the Heavens; owl; song of the birds; feather messages
The Ants and the Storm (page 75)	Big storm; cracks in the ground	Helping willow trees; leaf boats
The Rhythm Sticks (page 50)	Loud drumming; 'hurting' drum sticks	Golden weaver bird; rhythm sticks; music band
The Not-So-Perfect House (page 85)	Small door in the floor; hidden room; lock with no key	Large wooden chest; feathers; feather-covered bed; a good night's sleep
The Wombat Family (page 112)	Mother wombat's pouch; mother's milk in pouch	Mother's journey to find food; father wombat; digging claws; digging song; new tunnels

Story	Obstacles, hindrances, tempters	Helpers, guides
The Ocean Playground (page 117)	Long tentacles of octopus	Sea garden; little fish
A Family of Snails (page 142)	Journey to the bottom of the garden; leaving the snug flowerpot	Two homes: snug hole inside brick wall and snug flowerpot; moon shining bright; silvery trail
The Gnomes and the Golden Crowns (page 181)	Needy, greedy giant; dark cave	Song of the dragonfly; golden crowns; glass jar
Little Wolf (page 158)	Hunter's trap	Howling wolf song; wisdom of the wolf pack
The Boy and the Pearly White Shell (page 216)	Storm; loss of balance; fall into water; sinking deep	Pearly white shell; ocean singing a soft song
The Shy Robot (page 206)	Dusty top shelf; robber	Robot dance and song (in strong and clear rhyme)
The Barnacle-Covered Fish (page 222)	Cave in the reef; barnacles; 'Barnacle Bits' teasing song	Friendly lobster; rubbing dance
Clever Chameleon (page 88)	Strong elephant	Mole rat; hole in the ground
The Bowing Tree (page 115)	Famine in the land; greedy chief	The tree that bowed down; many fruits; the curious son
The Winged Horse (page 177)	Steep cliffs; dragon; black cave	Old wise woman; knife, flute and strand of silver hair; eggs and honey cakes; full moon; winged horse
The Rainbow Horses (page 171)	Separate colour groups; rainbow colour manes; grey clouds; flood	Warm caves; shining angel; weaving loom; golden horse; rainbow wings
The Digger that Always Says 'No'! (page 233)	Digger stuck on a negative rhyme (no movement)	Boy and girl enjoying playing in the sand; cup of tea (time to think)

Tips for choosing metaphors

Choose metaphors that directly relate to a particular behaviour

When writing a story for a specific behaviour, clues for metaphors for the main character can sometimes come from finding a corresponding animal, bird, insect or object with a similar quality – for instance a biting hippo (a flower or a butterfly would probably not work as a metaphor for biting!); a bashing crashing elephant (for hitting behaviour); loud banging drumsticks (for constant loud behaviour); a shy daisy (for withdrawn behaviour).

This can also work in reverse. For instance, in a story to help lead a child out of laziness and into work, you could begin the story about a lazy bee (the reverse or opposite of how a bee usually behaves) and then introduce some obstacles that it has to overcome, leading it into being a hard-working and happily creative bee.

Choose central metaphor from the child's favourite things (if possible and suitable)

When writing a story for a specific child, ideas for metaphors can be found by using the child's favourite animal or toy, or taking clues from her/his surrounding environment. Does the child have a passion for horses, for white rabbits, for dolphins, for trains? Does the child live by a river, in a forest or in a high-rise block in a city? What nature and/or daily experiences does the child have at home or at school that you could draw on for metaphor ideas?

Even knowing a child's favourite colour can help here. I learned this simple fact in my first year of teaching. I was desperately trying to find a way to come up with a story to address the behaviour of a five-year-old boy who always tried to blow out the story candle and push others off their chairs. I needed to find a way to engage his attention and help him settle down into a listening instead of a destructive mood. Then one afternoon his mother asked me if I knew where she could buy gold cloth – her son's birthday was next week and she said wanted to make him a gold cloak, adding that gold was his favourite colour. Taking this as a clue, I searched through my collections of folk- and fairytales and found a story that had a tree with a magic door in it that could only be opened by a golden key. I learnt the story and prepared to tell it the next week as a puppet show. I made a little golden key as a prop (cut from thick gold card) and hid it in a basket on my story table. During creative playtime I quietly took this boy aside and showed him where the key was hiding and asked if he would be my helper in the puppet show. I explained that I would need him to hold the basket during the story and pass me the golden key when it was time to open the magic door. For the first time since he had joined the group he sat transfixed during the story (with the little basket on his knee) and became engaged and attentive at story time from this day onwards. The golden key had opened more than the magic door in the tree!

I used a similar approach many years later when a child liked being a 'silly clown' during story time (trying to do headstands while all the other children were sitting listening). This child loved clowns so I found a story in which a goblin did many funny tricks (somersaults, headstands, etc.) and used a small doll to do these tricks in the puppet show. The child engaged fully with the puppet (and the story) and this seemed to break him out of this 'locked' behaviour, helping pull him into a listening mood at story time. Of course, during playtime, I gave this boy ample opportunity to do clown tricks!

Choose metaphors from class themes or content, or from child's own life

When writing a story for a whole group or class of children, clues for metaphors may be found from a theme in the curriculum or from the local school or home environment. Perhaps the class is studying history and the children are enjoying learning about knights in armour and brave deeds. A story for bullying could incorporate a magic (invisible?) shield or a crown of protection. Perhaps the children live in a town by the sea and have just explored the beach at low tide, finding an octopus to watch in a rock pool. Creative play time (at home or at school) is in need of an imaginative boost to help focus and settle a chaotic player – so the parent or teacher uses a story with ocean metaphors – an octopus with long tentacles that keeps knocking things over and a little fish that comes to the rescue.

Choose humorous or nonsense metaphors

When looking for clues for metaphors, there are no hard and fast rules – remember, stories don't fit comfortably with 'rules'! Sometimes humour can work very well. For example, in a story addressing over-excited and disruptive behaviour, the metaphor of 'an old red hat' (and a character like Panya the Rat who hides inside) slowly builds up a restless and disruptive mood as more and more animals come to live in Panya's house. The mood is beautifully soothed (in a funny, nonsense kind of way) when the final animal to come along is Hyena. Hyena sits on the hat and laughs a 'whooping' laugh because he thinks he is squashing all the friends. Meanwhile all the animals escape through a hole in the side of the hat, and Hyena is tricked. The movement of the story (and its metaphors) takes the listener into the disruptive experience and back out to a sense of calm and relief, through the simple use of humour and nonsense. A play made from this story could help strengthen therapeutic work.

Sometimes a story may catch the interest of a child because the metaphors are so removed from the originating situation. The story rhyme *A Day in the Life of my Hat* presents the image of a hat riding on a child's head like a rider on a horse: *When I play outside, my hat comes for a ride ... My head is the horse, pretending of course! ... My hat rides it around, as I run on the ground ... .* This makes a welcome and humorous change from the adult's constant nagging at the child to 'remember to wear your hat!'

Lateral thinking with metaphors

When choosing metaphors it helps to find ways to stretch your thinking. This requires playing with 'out of the box' ideas. With the above tips in mind, I suggest you make lists or mind maps, also called 'brainstorming', to help get many ideas down on a piece of paper – then begin to PLAY! You may be surprised by how the ideas take on their own life and build imaginative connections to each other.

A psychologist in Nairobi (I will refer to him as 'Mganga') worked this way on a story for a seven-year-old girl who at school had been acting out mature sexual behaviour. This girl's mother was a sex-worker – they lived in a little one-room shack, and the girl would watch the mother at 'work' then see the man leave money. Then mother would use money to buy food – so the child decided she wanted to earn money by imitating her mother's behaviour.

The main character for the story was an easy choice for Mganga. The girl used to come to the counselling session carrying a tattered old teddy bear, her only toy. He decided his story would be about a mother bear and a little bear. So at the workshop, 'bears' were put on his piece of paper. He had his starting point: *There was once a mother bear and a little bear and they lived in a small house in the forest.* But what metaphor could be used for the sexual activity? Many African animals were listed as a starting point ... then he had a flash of brilliance and chose the crocodile (or did it simply jump off the page at him?).

The crocodile required a river in the story. *There was once a mother bear and a little bear and they lived in a small house in the forest close to a river.* The mother bear, in order to get fish for little bear, needed to jump into a river full of snapping crocodiles to catch the fish. The hippopotamus was the next animal to 'jump up off the page'. After all, hippos also live in rivers in Africa. But Mganga wanted to use the hippo as a 'helper' and, feeling worried that this could be a little scary for the child, he looked for a better idea – a 'magic rock that looked just like a hippo's back'. This was the perfect helper needed to rescue the little bear when it also tried to jump into the river. The magic rock lifts the little bear out of the mother's working world (river full of snapping crocodiles), helps it safely back onto the river bank, and points it in the direction of the forest where honey and fruit (child-like food) were waiting to be gathered.

I will never forget the excitement in this particular workshop when Mganga shared his ideas. Then the whole group joined in and came up with a sequel idea – for use when the girl was older: the magic rock could help the little bear to make a canoe so it could safely cross the river and catch fish from a protected place (the group was divided on the significance of the canoe – some thought it was a metaphor for a condom, others thought it was a metaphor for protection in a wider sense, i.e. knowing how to say 'no'!)

Mganga didn't get a copy of his finished story to me in time to put in this book, but he reported in a phone call that he thought it had helped get a strong message to the girl about her still being a 'child'. This was all he had hoped for and a very worthwhile outcome.

Another example of lateral thinking happened in a group discussion about a story for a six-year-old boy who kept soiling his pants and was reluctant to sit on the toilet. The child loved the ocean, so, pursuing this line of thought, the group came up with the metaphors of a 'barnacle-covered fish' (for the soiled pants) and a cave (for the toilet). This fish was reluctant to go into the cave at the edge of the lagoon to learn the 'rubbing dance'. Eventually with the help of a friendly lobster he learnt the rubbing dance that helped to take off the barnacles that kept growing on his fishy skin. The fish could now swim freely in the lagoon with his friends (*The Barnacle-Covered Fish*, page 222).

Caution in choosing metaphors

At a workshop in Beijing (after my book had been published in China) a parent confessed to the group that he had tried to make a story for his three-and-a-half-year-old to encourage teeth cleaning. The story described little worms (germs) that, if they were not collected by the toothbrush, could come out at night to bite the teeth. Not surprisingly, the story scared his child, and the parent realized he should have used more transformative metaphors and resolution (perhaps the worms like swimming and need to be collected each night by the toothbrush then washed down the sink?) Or perhaps, for a child so young, he could have used a different kind of creative strategy for this situation (a teeth-cleaning song?) combined with active role modelling by the parents.

A story is definitely not appropriate if it is likely to scare the child. Stories should help make our children strong, and give them courage and understanding to face the future, but not frighten them!

The above confession generated a buzz of discussion – another parent shared a story she had used for her son who was always trying to dig into his ear to get out earwax (she had already taken him to a doctor to check there was nothing wrong inside the ear). In her story there was a wax rabbit that lived in the ear and it needed to sleep for a while then would jump out when it was ready. She realized after telling it (only once) that such a story could have given her boy nightmares … a rabbit is living in my ear! So the story wasn't used again. We discussed some alternative metaphors and eventually settled for a story about a fairy-sized leaf that would eventually fall off the 'ear tree' (inspired by the autumn leaves falling outside the workshop room window). The mother commented later about the effectiveness of such an approach – the boy had now stopped playing with his ear!

Another parent shared a story written for her daughter to encourage her to practise piano. In this story there was a music fairy that lived inside the piano and liked to dance when the piano was being played. However, this choice of metaphor 'backfired' as the daughter kept stopping her practice to open the piano and try to see the fairy dancing. On reflection, a different choice of metaphor would have been more effective – perhaps using an 'invisible' music fairy (emphasis on the 'invisible') who loved to dance around the room while music was being played. Of course, the age and stage of development of the child would need to be considered before trying to encourage such behaviour through creative storytelling (the discipline of piano practice might be regarded as more appropriate for an older child or teenager – see section on 'A question of ethics' page 28).

Building tension – the journey

> *Like pulling back the string on a bow before shooting the arrow, the greater the story tension (journey) the more directly the arrow (resolution/positive outcome) will reach the heart of the listener.*

The journey is the formative part of the therapeutic story structure. An eventful journey is a way to build 'tension' as the story evolves, and can lead the plot into and through the behaviour 'imbalance' and out again to a wholesome resolution. Stories for young children[9] usually only require simple events and small amounts of tension in the journey, whereas for older children events can be more detailed or complex, and supply greater tension as the journey unfolds.

The use of 'obstacle' and 'helping' metaphors is intricately connected with the journey. The tension or conflict (pulling back the string on the bow) in the journey is usually built up through the involvement of the 'obstacle' metaphors, and the resolution is achieved though the 'helping' metaphors.

When planning a therapeutic story journey, the following steps can be helpful once you have chosen your metaphors:

1: Decide what kind of 'movement' you want in your story:

- A story with a ***linear movement*** is one where the behaviour starts out of balance then comes back towards balance. For example, in the story of *The Rosella and the Strawberry Patch* (page 83) the Rosella is lacking confidence and independence; and then, through a sequence of events, gains confidence and independence.
- A story with a ***circular movement*** is one where the behaviour begins in balance, falls out of balance, then comes back towards balance. For instance, in the story of *The Singing Snake and the Dancing Bear* (page 212) the snake begins with a wonderful

singing voice then changes to using foul language to entertain the crowd in the circus; then, through a transformative sequence of events, finds his beautiful voice again.

2: Make notes on the 'bones' (summary) or the main sequences of the story – then add the 'flesh' (details). This approach makes it easier for you to play with ideas, and to change track if need be and rewrite your storyline. If you begin by writing every word down, you are less likely to be open to changing your ideas (even if they don't seem to be working) as you have already invested a lot of time in detailed writing. In another section of this book you will find some exercises to do with 'story bones' (on page 39).

However, in my own story-writing there have been times when I ignored both the steps above. Instead I might see a clear image (or a few images) in my imagination, already associated with obstacle and helping metaphors for my story journey. Then all I have to do is work on a word flow and 'flesh' out the storyline. This happened quite recently after a discussion with some Norwegian friends about the tragic events that occurred in their country in 2011, where many young people lost their lives in a shoot-out at an island camp. They mentioned the special Memorial Day that followed (a Rose March Tribute), where thousands of citizens gathered in Norwegian towns and cities, each carrying a single rose. In my mind's eye I saw the image of a long, sharp thorn that had grown in the wrong place on a rosebush. This thorn had pierced the heart of a beautiful rose and killed it, but many new roses were already growing up in the place where all the petals of the dying rose had landed. I didn't feel any need to play with the storyline, so simply sat down and wrote a story – *The Rose and the Thorn* (page 74 – for my friends' children's school in Arendal.

There are no hard and fast rules with any aspect of writing stories!

Different story journeys for different ages

Therapeutic stories, like folk- and fairytales, can be divided into 'categories of complexity'. In general, the gentler the theme or journey, the more appropriate the tale for younger children; the greater or more complex the difficulties or journey, the more appropriate the tale is for older children.

For a three- to four-year-old, the building of tension in the 'journey' can be as simple as using repetition of the same experience, or the repetition of a song or rhyme throughout the story. In the story of *Buddy Cuddle* (page 57), the grumbly children are taught magic words to get rid of the grumbly spell, and these magic words are repeated several times in the story to build the tension, as well as encouraging the listeners (the grumbly children) to use the words and movement of *stomp the ground and turn around* in real life:

Huff puff, gruff and stuff
Stomp the ground and turn around
Huff puff, gruff and stuff.

In *Little Siafu and her Shiny Stone Drum* (page 230), the safari ant begins by not wanting to be part of the group:

I'm tired of having to walk in line, I'm sick of having to keep in time,
I just want to sit in the sun, sit in the sun and play on my drum!

She tries to find new friends but when each new friend is not suitable, her dissatisfaction is repeated many times. The repetition of this little rhyme builds the journey tension.

Please go away and leave me be,
You are far too LOUD to play music with me.

After the children have heard it four times, they are thirsting for a positive solution, and longing for Little Siafu to find some friends as suitable playmates who are not too *LOUD, SLOW, FAST* or *BIG*. Eventually, Little Siafu realizes that she wants to be with her ant friends again and she starts singing a different tune:

I wish with my friends I could walk in line,
I wish with my friends I could keep in time,
I don't want to sit in the sun,
I want to walk with my friends and play on my drum!

Another way of building the tension is using repetition combined with a sequence of additional characters (often referred to as 'cumulative' stories). The repetition becomes the key structural device in the story by developing the action through a single, expandable image. The story of *Panya the Rat* (page 123) is an example here – a little rat finds an old hat then makes it his home; then along comes Chura the Frog and moves in with him; then along come several more animals, one by one, and they all move into the old hat. This build-up of characters makes the ending (the tricking of Hyena) more significant and powerful. There are other versions of this story from cultures around the world – e.g. 'Nibbler the Mouse', 'The Mouse and the Glove'. Without the build-up of characters, the story would simply be a recounting of a quite insignificant incident – 'A rat found an old hat and lived inside'.

In a story for an older child, the story 'journey' usually needs to be more involved, with a quest of some kind and several turning-points, set-backs or tasks along the road. In *The Winged Horse* (page 177), the twists and turns on the journey lead the listener deep into the story theme. If the boy had been granted his wish by the old woman whom he first visits in the forest, there would hardly have been a journey – the story would have finished too quickly, would have been too easy, would almost not have been a story (reflecting some modern situations where children's wishes are granted too quickly!). Instead the woman gives the boy three things – a sharp metal knife, a wooden flute and a strand of her long silver hair. The boy sets out on his quest, and with the help of the three gifts from the old woman he manages to climb the steep cliffs, tame the dragon and bridle and ride the winged horse.

To build resilience and strength of character, children today need to hear (and travel) these complex journeys – otherwise life can appear too easy and few powers of endurance are nurtured.

Examples of more complex journeys can be found in many of the well-known fairytales – such as 'Cinderella', 'Snow White', 'Rose White and Rose Red'. Some examples in this book include *The Bowing Tree, The Rainbow Horses,* and *Clever Chameleon*.

Writing the story journey is usually the most difficult part, but once you get some idea of the storyline – 'something out of balance comes back into balance' – and you have some ideas of one or more metaphors to work with, then at least you have a starting point.

To get a feel for the tension and journey in different stories (simple and complex), my advice to you is to read many children's stories. Try to borrow or buy collections of folktales from many different cultures. There are also many internet sites where one can access a wonderful range of stories.

The value of props

Some therapeutic stories are given extra strength by the use of a 'prop' or toy. Occasionally a therapeutic story lends itself to this strategy, but not always. Most have a storyline that carries the message quite simply on its own. However, some stories and situations have an obvious 'call' for props or puppets to be used in the telling, and then sometimes the prop(s) can be used by the child or children as a toy, or costume, or piece of jewellery after hearing the story.

Following an early morning robbery (involving theft and destruction) in a school in Nairobi, my colleague Silviah Njagi wrote *The Gnomes and the Golden Crowns* (page 181) for her class. Her aim was to give a message to the parents, the children and the teachers of how they could work together in rebuilding the kindergarten, giving them courage and confidence to face the future no matter what obstacles might appear! An obvious prop for each child (taken directly from the storyline) was a simple golden crown in the classroom made by finger-knitting threads of yellow-gold wool. Being able to wear these crowns – at school and at home (even to sleep in if need be) was a perfect idea for a strengthening story prop. There could also have been therapeutic value for the parents and teachers in helping the children make these props.

In the story of *The Wombat Family* (page 112) the mother reported that, to help the weaning process, she first told the story to her three-and-a-half-year-old, and then she used little stuffed wombats (a baby one, and two large ones for the mother and father) to help act it out. The child continued playing with the wombats, and the mother reported that at different times he asked some questions related to the story, like 'when baby wombat gets bigger, he doesn't milk any more, right?' The visual props seemed to help the story 'go in'. Similarly, with the story of *The Elephant's Trunk* (page 67), whether told at home or at school, it could be effective to use visual props to show how an elephant can use its trunk to lift something heavy. If a child or a group of children get to see the positive use of grandmother elephant's strong trunk pulling the little elephant to safety, this could help the storyline go in deeper.

After telling the story of *The Barnacle-Covered Fish* (page 222) for a six-year-old child who continually soiled his pants, it was suggested that the parent might sew a tiny felt fish for the child, all clean and new, just like the fish in the story. Perhaps it could be attached to a necklace for the child to wear, or stitched with a ribbon to be kept in the pocket of the child's jacket – a gentle reminder of the clean and happy (barnacle-free) fish.

Natalie, who contributed the toileting story of *The Gum Tree* (page 223) emailed me to describe how she had extended this storyline by using a toy wooden treehouse and some Gum Nut Babies. She writes that her three-year-old boy *loves these little toys so much, and we play with them together. I am able to role model any story or behaviour for him. It's been like magic watching him work out his fears or concerns through a simple propped story.*

Here is one of Natalie's examples of using props, following the success of *The Gum Tree* story:

> *My little boy was finding bath time a challenge – not being a fan of water nor wanting to get his face wet. Our night time story now has the Gum Nut Babies making their way home through the forest to their treehouse, to Mummy Gum Nut; and they go through a routine of coming home, going upstairs to the bathroom and having a lovely fun bath, then going up some more stairs to bed. The song the little Gum Nut Babies sing in their bath is:*
>
> *Rub a dub dub, Bubbles in the tub*
> *Splish splash splosh, Now it's time to wash*
> *Here and there … And now for our hair!*
>
> *It wasn't long after I introduced this story that my little boy stopped making a fuss about bath time and started to enjoy baths. Soon after this I even heard him singing in the bath, and the sound of pouring water, and I found that he'd picked up a cup and was washing his own hair with water pouring down all over his face. Now he'll stay in the bath for ages.*

Props can be used with a story in the following different ways:

- Giving the prop to the child as a gift to accompany the story
- Playing with props with your child while storytelling
- Telling the story to a group of children using props (as a puppet show)

None of these approaches mean one needs to buy something from a toyshop. There is magic and meaning in the use of simple home-made items … a stitched felt hat for a 'helping' elf or brownie; a painted wooden shield as 'protection' for a bullied child; a little star necklace to help overcome fear of the dark.

There is also magic and meaning in the use of simple objects found in nature … a pearly white seashell to help a noisy child learn to listen; some gum nuts or seedpods to use like little people in puppet shows; a shiny crystal as a good luck charm. I encourage you to collect props from nature both to inspire your storymaking and to use with your storytelling – seedpod boats, shells, nuts, acorns, feathers, driftwood, even a curl of wood shaving. The patterns, shapes and textures of the natural world offer unlimited ideas for story themes and story props.

A question of ethics

At the time of writing this book a probing question came to me in a workshop in Beijing – 'When is a story a healing story and when is a story manipulative?' The parent who asked the question then bravely continued by sharing that she was feeling guilty about a story she had recently made up. She had wanted to share a quiet meal together with her husband and asked her four-year-old daughter to watch TV in the next room. The daughter complained, saying that one of the cartoon characters was scary. The mother, taking an idea from the cow image printed on her daughter's T-shirt, made up a story about a cow protecting a child from being scared, and sent her back to the TV. Apparently the daughter came back to the parents after ten minutes saying, 'the cow is not helping!' and then (fortunately!) the TV was turned off and the child joined the parents at the table.

This example raises ethical questions and demands an examination of motives for writing stories for our children.

The *Oxford English Dictionary* definition of 'manipulative' (adjective), in relation to other people, is *exercising unscrupulous control or influence over a person or situation*. This is a marked contrast to the definition of 'healing' presented at the beginning of this chapter – *restore to health; bring into balance; become sound or whole*.

If we keep as our premise that therapeutic stories *help the process of restoring balance to an imbalanced behaviour or situation,* this gives us a clue to a **first question** to ask before writing our stories – i.e. is something out of balance in the first place? If not, then the chances are we could be trying to manipulate a behaviour or situation, not help or heal it. In the above example, there was nothing 'out of balance' with the child. It is perfectly natural for a child to be frightened by scary images on TV. What was out of balance was the motive of the parent, and fortunately, as she shared with the group, she now realized this and has learnt from the experience.

Similarly, a story created to encourage a child to 'jump' their appropriate stage of development, can fall into the 'manipulative' category (e.g. a story for bedwetting for a two-and-a-half-year-old; or a story to encourage intense study or music practice or sporting practice for a child too young to be able to cope with this). Usually they don't have any effect as the child is not developmentally ready to 'change', but I suggest that information on ages and stages of child development (physical, emotional, social, intellectual) should be researched by adults before sitting down to write 'healing' stories.

However, many stories for children, including cultural myths and fairytales, are written for general use, not specifically for a child whose behaviour is out of balance. The core values in such tales, usually some kind of change from an undesirable behaviour or situation to a more desirable one, have 'character building' purpose. They are therefore a valuable and ethical resource for parents and teachers as guides in helping to 'bring up' our children.

For this same reason, the stories in this book, although written for specific situations, can also have general use – the resolutions are transformational and invoke the child's own desire to change, the various undesirable behaviours have changed to more desirable behaviours, and the listener learns valuable character lessons from following these imaginative journeys.

For adults wanting to write stories for children, I suggest this is the clue to a **second question** to ask yourself before planning a storyline – 'Does the story encourage core values?' If the answer is yes, we know that it is not a manipulative story but a story to help guide children's development in a positive direction, not only for us but also for them.

Adjusting stories to different situations

As a story-maker, I like to keep alive the special stories that I find and write by sharing them with others. Sometimes a story might need to be adapted slightly for a specific situation.

If you find any example in this book that fits your situation but needs to be changed a little in places, please do use 'poetic licence' but strive to keep the integrity of the story. (Note: In my first book, *Healing Stories for Challenging Behaviour*, I have written in depth about the importance of preserving the story's integrity, especially where fairytales are concerned.)

Some of my stories in this book have been adapted from classic tales: *Hot Hippo* (page 95), *The Bowing Tree* (page 115) and *The Peddlar and His Caps* (page 139). Other examples of amended stories are discussed below.

Amended Wombat Story

A woman emailed me recently about a story for her son that helped encourage him to sleep in his own bed. She had attended the workshop in Singapore where a 'Wombat' story had been devised by her friend. Although this story had been written for a different purpose (to wean a three-and-a-half-year-old (see *The Wombat Family*, page 112) the mother thought that this story could also help with her situation (to wean an almost three-year-old from his parents' bed). So she made some small changes, shared it with her son, and wrote to me that 'It worked wonders for him!'

Another mother, wanting a weaning story for her three-year-old, changed the main character in the story from a wombat to a kangaroo – she emailed me that her daughter did not know about wombats but had started playing a little game where she would climb onto her mother's lap to drink milk and often called herself 'baby kangaroo', and her mother 'mama kangaroo'. As kangaroos also have pouches like wombats this was a perfect choice for this family situation.

One of my examples of amending stories to suit different situations is a 'doll' story that I first wrote for an orphan child called Silviah in the SOS children's village in Nairobi. I have since worked with and changed this story to suit two more situations: when a teacher passed away suddenly and we needed a story for her class (*A Doll from Heaven*, page 102); and for an orphan child who was bedwetting (*A Doll called Rainbow*, page 228).

Changing existing stories to suit different situations has two great advantages. Firstly it can be an easy road into a positive healing story experience, and secondly it can help give a taste for trying out more ideas. Amending an existing story is a stepping-stone experience to writing your own stories!

Changing story endings

A parent in a workshop shared an upsetting experience – her eight-year-old daughter was having nightmares from a story she had heard from her friends at school. It was about a clown that had stolen a baby out of its cradle while the babysitter was asleep. I mentioned this to my husband and he thought it might have come from a thriller movie about a clown. I contacted the parent later that day to suggest she try to rewrite the story with a positive/happy ending. I thought this could help relieve the daughter's nightmares. I even needed to make up an ending for myself to be able to sleep well that night!

A week later I received the following email:

Thanks for your idea of finding an ending to the clown story for my daughter Mali. I made up an ending about the clown being the uncle who works as a clown doctor at the local hospital. He had come home and entered through the back door; and when he heard the baby crying he picked her up to soothe her. Then they'd both fallen asleep in the next-door bedroom. When the parents came home all was revealed and it was a very happy ending. I told Mali that her friends had only told her half the story and that I'd since heard the ending. She had a few questions to test and make sure it did fit her story but she was generally really pleased to have that ending. It definitely seemed to ease her mind and take the terror out of the story for her.

This was such an interesting experience, and quite different (and easier) from writing a story from scratch – taking a scary story and rewriting the end – l think it could help many parents ...

The above example needs to be put in context. The eight-year-old girl had only heard half a story, which came from a thriller movie with a storyline inappropriate for her age group. The mother did her daughter a great favour in changing the ending.

This is very different from a child hearing a fairytale or a therapeutic story that has been devised with a healthy story journey and a positive resolution. There may be obstacles (even scary parts!) along the way, but these obstacles are overcome. If these were taken out there would be no obstacles to overcome, no positive progress!

On investigating children's stories through history and across cultures, one finds in every classic children's tale that there is either a simple problem to be solved, such as the peddler trying to get his caps back from the monkeys (*The Peddler and His Caps,* page 139) or a confrontation with evil that can take many forms, such as the hyena in the Kenyan version of *The Little Pigs and the Hyena* (page 183) or the witch in the Tanzanian tale *The Children and the Butterfly* (page 147).

In general, the milder a problem, the more appropriate the tale will be for younger children, while the greater the difficulties or the 'evil', the more appropriate the tale is for older children. But in all stories there is some degree of tension needed as an integral part of any story journey, whose different moods and challenges offer a kind of 'soul training' necessary for healthy child development. Modern 'sweet' or sentimental stories lack this quality of challenge. It may be tempting to avoid the stronger tales (where good eventually triumphs over evil) in an effort to protect our children, but to do so is to risk failure to develop sufficient capacities, later, for overcoming fear and bearing life's full reality.

The overriding rule here is the 'happy ending'. I believe we have a responsibility to find (or write) stories for children (especially younger ones) with journeys that overcome obstacles but always lead to positive, fair and happy endings.

Simplicity finds a way

As simple as a rabbit

An Indian mother in Nairobi, divorced but hoping soon to remarry, wanted to tell her four-year-old daughter about the marriage proposal from her new man. She chose to deliver the news in the form of a simple story about rabbits (her daughter's favourite animal). She told it at bedtime as a puppet show using toy rabbits and made the scenery with the bed blankets. The story was about a mother and child rabbit that had to say goodbye to father rabbit and find somewhere else to live. On their journey they met a new father rabbit who invited them into his house; the mother then asked her child, 'Do you think they should say yes, we will join you in your house?'

The mother's choice of story was very simple and quite direct. It was only one step removed from the real situation. But the good news was that it gained the result she was hoping for – the daughter apparently jumped up and down shouting 'yes' and wanted the story many times after this. You may think the mother took a risk (what if the daughter had said 'no'!), but perhaps she would have found a way to overcome this ... through another story?

I sometimes choose to use simple storylines when the situation and age of the child/children concerned doesn't seem to call for anything more complex – for instance in the story of 'Canoe Girl': *Canoe Girl is looking for a friend, a friend who would play with her and look after her*

... but where could such a friend be found? (page 169). This short story was written to help black children living in a predominantly white community develop a connection to their cultural identity via a dark-skinned doll. (In a predominantly black community this story could be reversed for white children.) This story idea came from the 'Cloud Boy' story that I had written for my own son (see *Healing Stories for Challenging Behaviour*). Although extremely simple, it had a powerfully positive effect on my son and our family situation.

Other examples of simple stories in this book (that almost totally ignore my suggested framework!) are *The Shining Star* (page 185), *Rainbow Colours* (page 90) and *The Lonely Robin* (page 207). What counts is that all three of these stories achieved a therapeutic effect.

The proof of the pudding is in the eating; the proof of the therapeutic story is in the behaviour change that follows the telling!

Such a simple straightforward format is not always effective as it only provides a brief imaginative journey for the listener. But ... sometimes it *can* be effective! Never underestimate the power of simplicity!

As simple as a 'strawberry poem'

A parent once came to me in a workshop with a challenge – how to stop her four-year-old boy eating all the strawberries in the strawberry patch before they were ripe? She found the task of writing a story too great, so I encouraged her to work on a poem. She put together the following poem that she later reported had worked well (the unripe strawberries were left intact!). In fact the poem became part of a daily chant when the family went out into the garden.

> *Strawberry, strawberry, your cape will soon be red,*
> *I shall help to make you a bed*
> *With warm dry straw like the forest floor,*
> *And soil so sweet, to bury your feet,*
> *Strawberry, strawberry, soon spring will be here,*
> *The time for eating is very near!*

In the spirit of simplicity, I have included several 'therapeutic' poems in this book (not counted in the 101 stories). You will find them scattered like daisies in the grassy carpet of stories – e.g. *The Stick that Sings* (page 55), *A Day in the Life of my Hat* (page 107), *Little Polar Bear* (page 209), and *Seasons* (see page 168).

Sometimes a poem can hold all you need to say!

Healing stories for all ages

Caterpillars, rabbits, gazelles, dolphins and hidden bullets

Stories don't like to be fixed in an age box. Sometimes a story written for a child may have a transformative effect on an adult. This is usually unplanned and sometimes subtle, sometimes strong.

I once wrote a simple nature story for young children about a little zebra that was brown and white (like all young zebras), but this little zebra wanted to grow up quickly and become black and white. The little zebra tried several ways to change his brown stripes to black ones (rolling in black mud, rubbing against a fire-blackened tree stump, even standing in the shade) and eventually gave up trying. Then he joined his friends playing and eating on the grassy plains and began to enjoy being a little zebra. I put this story in the weekly newsletter published by the school in Nairobi where I was working. A few days later, a parent who had been attending my parent education classes, rushed up to me in the school car park in a very excited mood. 'I have just read your story about Little Brown Zebra,' she said. 'Now I get it – our children need time to have a childhood!'

Some other examples, with quite strong effects, are discussed in the preliminary notes of some stories in this book, including *The Three Pots* (page 121) and *The Not-So-Perfect House* (page 85).

Stories for adults

Quite apart from the unplanned effects of children's stories on adults, however, sometimes an adult has an urgent need to write a story specifically for their own adult situation. I often experience this in my workshops, and I am continually surprised and delighted at how my framework for writing stories can be used for all ages. Even though this book is about healing stories for children, it seems important to briefly address this therapeutic approach for adults.

A poignant example happened at a workshop south of Sydney a few years ago. When I was compiling a list of 'challenging behaviour' for small-group story-writing, a mature woman put up her hand to make a contribution. She said she would like to work on a story for a three-year-old who had been sexually assaulted by a stranger in a park. A few other participants felt moved to join her writing group, and when it came time to present their story, they shared *The Caterpillar* (page 199). The woman then confessed to the whole group that the story was for her own situation, and thanked her small-group members for their contribution and support. She acknowledged that since this experience happened to her at the age of three, she had carried an 'isolated/disconnected' feeling all her life. She felt she had revisited the issue at an emotional and psychological level but this story about *The Caterpillar* helped her at to accept the experience at a deeper level without having to understand it. As the large group sat listening in awe and amazement, she described how the story imagery and the altered point of view brought new layers of meaning to her life, and a sense of wonder and transformation.

Another poignant situation happened in Nairobi when I was running a workshop for Médecins Sans Frontières (Doctors without Borders). Alongside the 30 or more therapists/counsellors there were some HIV patients who also wished to attend. At the morning tea-break a young man came up to me and told me that he didn't have much longer to live and that he wanted to write his life story. He asked if he could work on it during the workshop. Of course I said yes, and then for the rest of the day I observed him in a corner with a pen in hand, writing away on a pad held up close to his face (his eyesight was failing). At the end of the workshop I sat with him while he read his story – he had chosen to write about the life of a rabbit family. He said that choosing the rabbit metaphor had given him the freedom to express what had really happened – he felt free to describe how his father had beaten his mother (he didn't have to refer to his real father, but could tell a story about a father rabbit), how his mother had died an HIV victim, and how he had then left home to live on the streets (in the story – 'out alone in the fields'). His story had a touching ending, as he was found and taken in by another rabbit family (Médecins Sans Frontières) which gave him much love and care.

Another example of an adult story came from a young woman who wanted to overcome her 'timidity' in the workplace. She wrote a story about a jungle full of animals and a tiger (bully) that was out to catch them. In the story the shy gazelle, with the help of the silver moonlight, set a trap and caught and overcame the tiger.

On a lighter level, a situation that sometimes presents itself is when a participant desperately wants a story to help improve a challenging domestic situation – a story to 'change' the outlook of their husband or wife. I don't have any results to present here (sorry!), but I know that some have found it a cathartic experience to devise such stories. An example that comes to mind was when a young wife wanted a story to help motivate her husband to wash the dishes each night – she worked on a story that brought the dishes to life: oh how they longed for other hands to touch them! I am sorry that I never found out what effect such a story had, but her sharing of the 'story bones' (the basic narrative structure – see section below on 'Story bones') brought much laughter to her and to the group at the end of a long day.

Healing stories for teenagers

I have had several experiences of how this healing story framework can help teenagers. This has happened indirectly through my work with counsellors or psychologists, and it has usually involved a variety of powerful, unique and subtle story journeys. On one occasion a story resonated strongly with a sixteen-year-old indigenous Australian girl who had attempted suicide several times; and the message was strengthened by the gift of a pearl necklace to the girl. I later heard that the story had helped improve her self-esteem by giving her the sense she had something good and beautiful to hold onto. I didn't get a copy of the full story, but the 'story bones' (see section below) were as follows: *Girl on beach – falls asleep in sun – dreams of a dolphin (her indigenous totem) – dolphin is in trouble – dolphin is being sucked down – the more it fights the pull of the water the more it is being sucked into deeper and deeper, blacker and blacker water – then realizes it is trapped in oil spill – blacks out and floats to surface and is washed up on beach – girl wakes up and finds a shining pearl lying in the sand – puts pearl on a string and wears it around her neck – pearl becomes her protector.*

Choices of metaphor here require 'out of the box' thinking. For a 14-year-old Chinese girl whose parents had divorced (and neither of them wanted her to live with them) a therapist used a story of 'the gunnan orange' – a fruit in China that is famous for its sweet taste. In the story the orange falls off the train on its way to market and lands in a deserted patch of weeds – at first the orange thinks its life has been wasted but then it finds the strength in one of its seeds to 'grow again'.

Another example, this time of a story with many chapters, was written by a psychologist together with his client, a seventeen-year-old boy who had been driving a car that crashed into a tree and killed three of his friends (all extremely intoxicated). Called *The Hidden Bullet,* the story idea was conceived by the psychologist during one of my workshops, and the process of writing each chapter evolved slowly during therapy sessions with the boy.

The story was about a captain that led his soldiers into battle. All the soldiers were killed but he survived, with one bullet wound so deep that no doctor could find the bullet. The captain returns home and goes on a quest to find and transform this 'hidden bullet' (representing guilt and self-hate). The quest involved many tasks, including visiting and serving the families of his friends … both in the story and in real life.

The healing power of story has no bounds!

2

Getting the Story Juices Flowing

More and more today I meet people who are thirsting for imaginative approaches, in all professions and walks of life, to balance the domination of the intellectual and rational approach in most modern teaching and learning systems. Most of us are like 'dried-up prunes' and need stories and metaphors that can transform our imagination into juicy plums.[10]

In our busy adult lives, it is easy for our imaginations to 'dry up'. Like a muscle, the imagination can atrophy from lack of use and may need exercises to build it up again. Most primary and secondary learning is centred in the sciences and rational thinking – this was certainly the case in my education, and largely continues today. I recently listened to a radio interview with a young 'Nobel laureate' who had won his award in the field of mathematics. This young man acknowledged that when he was at school, even though he was brilliant in mathematics and science, his creative skills were almost non-existent. He commented how he wished he had been given a more imaginative education! As an example of the lack of expressive creativity in his childhood, when asked to write a story about 'home' he had listed every item in each room of the house, and then counted them!

Our creativity can be stimulated first by reading and then by attempting to write stories and poetry. If your imagination feels like a 'dried-up prune', my suggestion to you is to start by choosing ten stories in this book and reading one each day. Although these stories are written primarily for children, you may find the metaphors and imaginative journeys feed your adult soul. If this is of benefit, I suggest you continue reading more short stories … folk- and fairytales from many cultures, nature stories, funny stories, tall stories. There are so many genres of stories that can nourish your imagination. Fantasy novels and trilogies like *The Lord of the Rings* are another rich source of creative nourishment. It may also help to participate in a storytelling or writing course, and attend storytelling sessions.

Mother Nature can be a wonderful source of inspiration for the adult imagination. When I am pondering ideas for a story, I find some of my best ideas in nature. Walking through forest or bushland, or along the beach, sitting in the park or in the garden – these experiences have fed my imagination when I had 'writer's block'. Nature can refresh, cleanse, strengthen and nurture us. Especially if I am writing stories for young children, to be really open in heart and mind I find I need to bathe in the wonder and beauty of nature on a regular basis.

'Story bones'

The exercises in the story section of this book, at the end of each 'behaviour category' may help you create your stories. Called 'story bones', they give a summary or the 'bones' of a storyline and leave the reader free to fill in the details, work on a word flow, and turn into a finished narrative.

Many of the ideas for these 'story bones' have been taken from workshop discussions. Each one includes the outline of a story journey to which you can add metaphoric 'clothes' to flesh it out. Some are very brief, some have been partly completed, and some include several options for possible storylines and possible endings.

These exercises can help even the most experienced story-maker. Recently, my step-daughter Evie loaded a plea on Facebook – *Not enjoying my three-and-a-half-year-old's 'No – I don't want to' stage … very frustrating! Time to get creative I think, any tips?* I was in Kenya at the time and felt motivated to write a story. I sat at my laptop wondering where to begin, then I remembered that the 'story bones' exercises I was planning in this book included one called *The Digger that Always Says No!* The original story idea had come from a workshop in Sydney – the group wanted a creative approach for an uncooperative four-year-old who said 'no' to everything. They had come up with a simple outline and a little rhyme: *The digger says no, so nothing can grow!* I took these story bones and filled it out to finish the story (see page 233), including a few things that were personal to my grandson Harrison – his love of strawberries, digger machines and playing in the sand pit. Within a day the story was emailed to Evie and she enthusiastically turned it into a picture book for Harrison's daily story-time.

I am hoping these story bones exercises at the end of each story section will offer an easy springboard into your own story-writing. However please remember that they are suggestions only. The stories could be written with many different choices of metaphor and journey. Feel welcome to email me your finished story with a description of how it helped a challenging situation or behaviour … perhaps it could be used in my next book, creating a lively circulation of stories round the globe!

Imagination exercises

As well as attempting the 'story bones' exercises mentioned above, here are a few more ideas to help get the imaginative juices flowing.

Start with a children's song or nursery rhyme … then develop it into a story. This exercise is a very good way in to story-writing, and you will be surprised how easy it is to make up simple stories this way, especially for very young children.

Example: 'Here we go round the Mulberry Bush' (popular children's song/game)

Mrs (or Mr?) Mulberry lived in a little round house under a large mulberry bush. One morning she decided it was time to wash the curtains. She reached up high and one by one took the curtains off their hooks (make up song or rhyme here, and sing it to the Mulberry Bush tune – this is the way we take down the curtains; or, 'one by one, off the hook, one by one, hook by hook'). Then she filled the tub with soap and water and started to rub ('This is the way we wash the curtains, squeeze the curtains, rub the curtains … ' etc.). When the curtains were washed and squeezed, Mrs Mulberry carried them out to the line and reached up high to peg them on ('This is the way we peg them up, one by one, peg them fine, one by one, along the line') etc., etc. This story could carry on for much longer, following the process of the sun and wind drying the clothes; then Mrs Mulberry unpegs the curtains and brings them inside, irons them, then hangs them back up.

A story like this could have therapeutic value if, for example, a child's favourite toy needed to be washed and the child was reluctant to let it go. The teddy or doll could be added into the story of Mrs Mulberry's washing-day, or used in exchange for the curtains, giving a picture of the cycle of washing and drying.

Example: 'Incy Wincy Spider' (popular nursery rhyme/ action rhyme)

One morning, Incy Wincy spider decided he wanted to see more of the world, so he left his home under the bushes and walked across the garden … (use a walking song or rhyme?). Then he reached the wall of a house and climbed up the water spout (use first part of Incy Wincy rhyme here ×2). Then he walked across the roof … (walking song?). Then a strong wind came and blew some rain clouds over the garden and the rain washed Incy Wincy off the roof, back down the water spout, roly-poly, roly-poly, roly-poly, all the way to the ground. Once on the ground he quickly ran back to his home under the bushes, glad to be safe and cosy again. Later that day the sun came out and dried up all the rain, so Incy Wincy spider climbed up the spout again!

A story like this could be used on a walk when a child or group of children get upset about being caught in the rain – perhaps the teacher or parent has to spend time under shelter with the children and could fill in the time with a little – or long – story about 'Incy Wincy'. This would keep the children occupied and at the same time help reassure any anxieties with knowledge that 'The sun will shine again.'

Some examples of stories in this book that have been constructed from and inspired by existing rhymes and songs are *The Shouting Clock* (page 218), *Little Siafu and Shiny Stone Drum* (page 230) and *The Little Drummer Boy* (page 173).

I encourage you to choose some of your children's favourite rhymes or songs and turn them into little stories – it can be a most satisfying process. The story can just be fun and enjoyable – there is great value in this! Or you may find a way to link this exercise to a therapeutic need – for instance, if your child is a fussy eater and you are trying to encourage her/him to try new foods (eggs for breakfast?), a story about Humpty Dumpty could help. You could even use poetic licence and change the ending: perhaps Humpty did get fixed so he could be taken to market to be sold to a little child for breakfast. Or maybe he fell off the wall into a frying pan and got scrambled … Such a story would fall into the category of 'Nonsense stories' – a genre for children that adults must be careful not to take too seriously. They speak to a child's budding sense of humour, and even defy the golden 'happy ending' rule for stories for young children. The very nature of nonsense implies 'no rules'.

For stories for older children, one can find inspiration in ballads: *The Highwayman, Hiawatha, The Butterflies' Ball and the Grasshoppers' Feast,* or *Waltzing Matilda.* One of our classic Australian movies was a story made from a bush ballad of the same name – *The Man from Snowy River*. Funny and nonsense poems can be another source for ideas. To name just a few: *They Went to Sea in a Sieve; The Owl and the Pussycat; Wynken, Blynken and Nod*.

Make nature observations and collect natural props that suggest story ideas … the patterns, rhythms and metaphors in the natural world can offer a wellspring of ideas for therapeutic story-making.

Example one

Observations in my spring/summer Australian garden led to my story of *The Frangipani Gift*, a soothing story for four- to six-year-olds about waiting, and patiently taking time. Mother Nature gave me all I needed here for a story to settle a rather restless class, combined with a story to suit our Australian summer-Christmas mood. The busyness in my spring garden – bees, butterflies, flowers bursting out everywhere – contrasted with the quiet waiting of the frangipani flower that doesn't come to bloom till just before Christmas.

In the story, the flower children, the bees and the butterflies (all in turn) dance around the brown bare branches of the frangipani tree, calling:

Frangipani Child – Come out, come out, to dance and play,
Springtime is here and the world is bright and gay.

But still the Frangipani Child keeps sleeping, and the wind whispers to the flower children:

Frangipani is waiting for a special time,
Frangipani is waiting for a golden light to shine.

Finally that special time comes (see page 131 for the whole story) – by which time the restless class had settled into such a quiet mood that one could almost hear the frangipani flower opening! All were waiting to hear what this special time might be.

Example two

A listening game I like to play with groups of children (ages three to eight) involves passing a large shell around the circle to a song – *Shell, shell, you must wander, from one beach to another; oh how beautiful, oh how beautiful, shell where are you now?* I am continually surprised how even the noisiest child will quietly wait so they can have a turn to hold the shell and listen to the sound of Mother Ocean.

When I was asked to write a story for a 'noisy' nine-year-old, who, according to his teacher, could never stop talking, I thought immediately of involving a shell in the story and wrote *The Boy and the Pearly White Shell* (page 216). The story takes the child deep down into the quiet of the ocean depths, where he finds a pearly white shell that leads him back to the surface (and saves his life). From this time on, the boy carries his pearly white shell with him wherever he goes. He has a velvet bag to keep it in, and every day he takes his shell out of the bag and holds it up to his ear and listens ... he can hear the ocean singing a soft song of how the pearly white shell saved his life.

> Tell memory stories ... they can have simple yet surprising therapeutic value and are another easy pathway into storytelling.

While writing this book I had some challenging experiences babysitting two children (a girl aged five and a boy aged seven). I was finding it difficult to settle them down one night as, no matter what I did, they continued to fight and argue. Finally it was bedtime and even from their beds they were still at odds with each other; so I decided to tell them a story from my own childhood.

I gained their attention by pure accident, as, trying to avoid their arguments about what story they did or didn't want, I told them 'I'm not going to tell a story – I am going to do something different'! Then I shared with them one of my most special childhood memories ... which I called *Saturdays* (see page 145). They both seemed soothed as I recounted this harmonious adventure which my brother and I experienced every Saturday when we were young. The next babysitting night I was met at the door with cries of 'Can we have another one of those *different* stories?'

Memory stories are another pathway into storytelling and storywriting, and each one of us has a treasure chest of stories unique to our own lives and surprisingly interesting to young ears!

My seven-year-old grandson Tosh reached a stage where he was trying to piece together family connections. At first he found it quite difficult to understand that I used to be married to his father's father, as he only had known me as 'sho-sho' (Kikuyu for 'grandmother') and as John's wife! To help him with this, I began telling him stories about the times when Nigel (his grandfather) and I were hitching around the world in the 1970s and stories of family experiences when his father was a young boy. He was intently interested (more so than in any of my other stories) and he continued for quite a while asking for 'true' stories every time we were together.

One of the contributors to this book, Natasha Hund, re-affirms this therapeutic value of memory stories. The sharing of family memory stories in *Big Things When You are Little* (page 144) has been an effective way of easing anxiety in her separated family situation. Natasha writes that *through stories I wanted to connect my daughter to some of our childhood memories, and bring a sense of unity. With her father not present in the household I used stories to keep his presence alive outside the times she spent with him.*

> *Create your own Story Bag or Story Box (an old chest perhaps). Any intellectual thought or planning is taken away as you dip into the bag or box with your eyes closed to choose several items that will form your story … an exercise in pure imagination!*

Take a bag or a box and fill it with all kinds of interesting items. These are used to 'spark' the story … a golden feather, a glass marble, a pearl necklace, a silver ring, a bright shiny penny, a smooth pebble, a shell, an old key, some toy figurines (people, animals, birds, fish, insects, etc.), small musical instruments, a miniature teapot, a strip of blue velvet, some see-through gauze, some shells and seedpods and other props from nature … the list could be endless.

Second-hand stores are a great source of items for the 'story box' – a hand mirror, gloves, old medicine bottles, old buttons, old Christmas ornaments, different fabric scraps …

It seems just about anything will trigger a memory or spark an idea for somebody.

You can choose to work with this exercise on your own; or gather a group of people together: one person pulls out a pre-determined number of items from the box (I suggest no more than three) and gives them to the next person, who has to make up a short story in which those things somehow come into play.

It can be helpful to set parameters for this exercise, such as time/place/season etc. Especially if one is aiming to work on a therapeutic story, the age group of the listeners would be an important aspect.

Another fun kind of game is to sit in a circle with a group of family members or friends or colleagues and pass round the 'story bag' or 'story box' – each adult picks out an item and they must somehow use it to move the story forward. This may not end up with a well-formed story (though it might!) – but it involves a group in the shared creative activity of story-making, stimulating each person's imaginative capacities in a supportive context. It is also just plain fun!

The 'Story Bag' story

I can't mention the 'story bag' without paying tribute to my Xhosa friend from South Africa, Nomangesi Mzamo Mbobosi, who passed away in February 2011. Nomangesi was one of the pioneers of teacher training work in the slums outside Cape Town when I was working in South Africa. We were both employed by the CCE (Centre for Creative Education). I met her in 1996 and involved her as a 'critical friend' in my cross-cultural research project. Nomangesi was a great storyteller and shared many wonderful stories with me. Indeed, her life was an amazing story – of courage, determination, resilience and generosity. I feel privileged to have known her and her stories. She survived terrible apartheid experiences and always sustained her hope for South Africa to be a true rainbow (multicultural) nation.

Nomangesi nurtured my fledgling connection with Africa with her open perspective on having a 'white Australian' as a teacher of storytelling to African students. In her own words:

Forget that you are a white Australian and think of yourself as a human educator sharing stories world-wide – you have been sent here by God. This is your task – children are born with treasures in their hands. You are someone who has a key to open these treasures through stories.[11]

In the training courses in Cape Town I was helping teachers make story bags to fill with story props. These bags were to hang on a hook in the corner of their shack kindergartens – as most of their small classrooms did not have the luxury of storage shelves. Nomangesi was working as my interpreter. She was inspired by these craft ideas and came up with an idea for a Story Bag song and Story Bag story and told it to my groups of students (I have put her oral telling into written words for this book). I believe her choice of metaphors was very close to her real-life experiences – the 'strands of slimy seaweed' reflecting the desolate slum areas of her home, and the 'story treasures' reflecting her enduring hope for the future of South Africa.

'Story Bag' Xhosa song

Umama ntlanzi, umama ntlanzi, Ufunubutyebi, ufunubutyebi, Ubutyebi babantwana (×2), Abantwana bakhe (×2).

Ubutyebi ngamabali (×2), Abantwana Bakhe (×2).
(Mother Fish is looking for treasures, treasures for her children –
the treasures are stories)

'Story Bag' story

There was once a Mother Fish who cared for many little children.
This Mother Fish wanted to find beautiful treasures for all her family,
and so she searched the ocean floor for the shells and white pearls
that she had heard Mother Ocean singing about. But no matter how
long and hard she looked, she wasn't able to find beautiful treasures
anywhere – the part of the ocean where she lived only seemed to have
old strands of slimy seaweed and rough stones on the sandy bottom.

Mother Fish decided to go to the Wise Old Turtle who wandered
the ocean worlds and knew all the secrets of the sea. When she found
Old Turtle she told him the problem.

After thinking for a long time, Old Turtle said: 'You can turn what
you have into treasures if you do as I suggest. Gather up some seaweed
and weave it together to make a strong bag. When it is finished, put
many little stones into the bottom of the bag, and then drag the seaweed
bag to the top of the water where the golden rays of sunlight shine down.
Catch some of this golden light and then close the bag tightly and take it
back home with you and leave it closed for three days. When you open
it, then you will find beautiful treasures for your children.'

Mother Fish did as Old Turtle said. It took a long time to gather
the seaweed and make the bag, and then with the stones inside it was
hard work dragging it to the top of the ocean where the sunlight shone
in, and then it was also hard work dragging it back down to her home
once she had caught some sunlight and closed the bag tight.

Of course, when she returned home, all her children swam around
the bag wondering what could be inside. For three days it stayed closed,
and then when Mother Fish opened it – what do you think she found?

The golden light had worked a magic spell on the stones and
turned them into story gems – hundreds of beautiful story treasures
for her children. And from that day on Mother Fish told stories to
her children from the story treasure bag, and there could not have
been a more wonderful gift to give them.

The old turtle had indeed been very wise!

Section B
101 Therapeutic Stories

This section spans a collection of 101 stories for commonly identified forms of challenging behaviour or other challenging situations. To help you find your way, the pages are organized into the following sixteen categories with suggested stories for diverse possibilities. These categories have been chosen as easy reference, but it is certainly not recommended that they be used as 'labels' for behaviour.

- Anger/Aggression/Hitting/Scratching/Biting
- Anxious/Insecure/Fearful
- Bullying/Exclusion/Teasing
- Death/Dying/Illness
- Disrespect/Lack of Care (self/others/things)
- Disruptive/Restless/Over-excited
- Dishonest/Sneaky
- Divorce/Separation/Blended Families
- Fussiness/Complaining
- Intolerance/Lack of Acceptance (of self and others)
- Lack of Confidence/Resilience
- Sexual Abuse/Sexual Awareness
- Shy/Withdrawn/Low Self-esteem
- Swearing/Shouting/Silly Speech
- Toileting/Bedwetting
- Obstinacy/Lack of Social Sense

The 101 stories include some from contributing writers, some from my own writing collection and some transcribed from traditional folk- and fairytales. Some stories have already been used (with different degrees of success) and have notes documenting their use. Others have been newly written or transcribed for this book. Any correspondence from the use of these stories and/or any of your own therapeutic stories is welcome – www.healingthroughstories.com

The stories are mainly suitable for children aged from three to ten, although some have been used successfully with teenagers and adults. Each story is preceded by notes indicating suggested ages and usage.

Story bones

Each category of stories includes the 'bones' of one or more story ideas. These 'story bones' have been included as story-making exercises for you, the reader. Most of these have come from workshop discussions. Each one includes the outline of a story journey for you to flesh out and complete if you wish with metaphoric 'clothes'. These are suggestions only. The stories could be written with many different choices of metaphor and journey.

These stories are only a few drawn from a story well that contains inexhaustible resources. With the help of the first section in this book on Writing Therapeutic Stories, it is my hope that you will explore many more ideas.

Reading or telling

The choice between telling or reading these stories to your child or children is left up to you. Unless it comes naturally to you, storytelling usually requires more effort as the adult has to learn the story first, but some 'stepping stones' can help here: telling some parts and reading others; drawing pictures of story sequences while telling; or using puppets in storytelling (see Section 5 of *Healing Stories for Challenging Behaviour* for different ways of preparing and learning stories, and using props and puppets to help in the telling). The wonderful oral tradition of telling stories creates more direct contact between teller and listener, since there is no book intervening in the story experience. Maureen Watson, an indigenous Australian storyteller, says that told stories 'touch' the audience in a different way. I have experienced this many times – through eyes, voice and gestures the storyteller weaves invisible threads with listeners, and can 'hold' them from start to finish. This 'holding' power of storytelling can help develop and strengthen concentration, and hence increase the child's capacity for learning. In her book *Storytelling with Children*,[12] Nancy Mellon offers fine insights into the value and power of this process.

Although the 'telling' experience is undoubtedly a more lively and personal way of sharing a story, both telling and reading are important ways of delivering or presenting stories. There is a place for both. Especially with the dominance of 'screen' media in children's lives today, having stories told and/or read by adults is a wonderful blessing. Sometimes, especially in one-to-one situations, the 'book' can be a bridge for the story sharing, bringing a sense of closeness through sitting side by side, or with a young child on the adult's lap.

If you choose to work with a particular story from this book, an option is to turn it into a picture book using your own (or the child or children's) illustrations, then read from this newly created story-book.

3

Anger/Aggression/Hitting/ Scratching/Biting

The Rhythm Sticks

This story idea came from a group workshop in Nairobi in response to the need for a therapeutic strategy for a six-year-old boy who was continually hitting others. The use of the drum and rhythm sticks seems a perfect metaphor for the 'hitting'. The story offers a transformation from 'hitting for hurting' to 'hitting for playing'. At the end of the story I have included three music games that I have used for many years with groups of children, aged from two (playgroup) to eight years.

There was once a town famous for its musical fairs. In this town lived a boy who loved to beat the drum. This boy wanted to join the band that played at the fair.

Bim-bam, bim-bam, bim-dam dum, this is how I beat my drum!

But the boy was always playing too loud and too fast – he was always beating his drum too hard and too fast – and he didn't get chosen for the band.

Feeling angry and upset, the boy kicked a hole in his drum, left the fairground and walked into the forest. Oh he was angry! He was so angry he started to hit the trees with his drum sticks.

Bim-bam, bim-bam, bim-dam dee, this is how I beat the tree!

Oh he was angry! He was so angry he started to hit the rocks with his drum sticks.

Bim-bam, bim-bam, bim-dam dock, this is how I beat the rock!

Soon the boy grew tired of hitting trees and rocks. He tried to hit out at a butterfly that was flying by, but fortunately the butterfly changed direction just in time! He tried to hit out at a frog that was hopping by, but fortunately the frog changed direction just in time! He tried to hit out at a tortoise that was sleeping near the path, but the tortoise had such a strong hard shell that he didn't seem to notice – he just kept on sleeping.

Then a golden weaver bird flew in front of the boy. The weaver had some sticks in its mouth. The boy watched as the weaver reached its nest and used the sticks to weave into its tree house. The boy was amazed by the skill of the bird and started to play his drumsticks to the rhythm and movement of the bird working its weaving.

Rickity-tick, rickety-tick, rickety-tick, I click my sticks.

After a while, the boy left the weaver to finish its nest, and he returned through the forest. As he walked along the path, he continued to play the weaver-bird rhythm:

Rickity-tick, rickety-tick, rickety-tick, I click my sticks.

As he came closer to the fairground, the band-leader heard him coming. This is just what we need in our band, thought the band-leader, and he invited the boy with his rhythm sticks to join the rest of the musicians.

Rickity-tick, rickety-tick, rickety-tick, I click my sticks.

At the town fair that year, the boy played beautiful music with his rhythm sticks on-stage with the band. He continued to practise his music, and for his next birthday he was given a new drum. Now he was able to make beautiful music with his rhythm sticks and with his drum.

Rat-a-tat, rat-a-tat, rat-a-tat tum, this is how I play my drum!
Rickity-tick, rickety-tick, this is how I click my sticks.
Rat-a-tat, rickety-tick, I play my drum and click my sticks.

There once was a boy who played his body drum

A hand and finger rhyme that can be chanted as a poem or put to music, and can be repeated several times with 'boy', 'girl', 'teacher', 'mother', 'father', etc.

There once was a boy who played his body drum
Rat-a-tat, rat-a-tat, rum-a-tum-tum.
He played on his knees to make a body drum
Rat-a-tat, rat-a-tat, rum-a-tum-tum.
Sometimes his elbows, and sometimes his hands,
Rat-a-tat, rat-a-tat, rum-a-tan-tan.
He played on his toes and he played on his head
Rat-a-tat, rat-a-tat, rum-a-ted-ted.
This little boy loved to play his body drum,
Rat-a-tat, rat-a-tat, rum-a-tum-tum.

Who wants to play on the great big drum?

This music game can be chanted as a poem or put to music. The game will need a drum – either a real drum (an African jembe is perfect for this), or a pumpkin, or an upturned tin. If playing this with a large group of children, you could choose two children at a time, then sing both names – e.g. 'Katie and Jason want to play on the great big drum' followed by 'They can play it loudly' etc.

Who wants to play on the great big drum?
Katie wants to play on the great big drum.
Katie can play it loudly,
Katie can play it softly,
Katie can play it very fast,
Katie can play it slowly.

I step and step and step

This is a joyous music game I was taught many years ago when I was training to be a teacher (in 1976!). It is a great one to use at morning ring time – every child is given an instrument and then the teacher leads them round the circle, doing the actions as the children play the instruments. I have used this with instruments as simple as seedpods (for shaking) and sticks (for clapping together). The children very quickly learn how to be careful when making music – the rule, of course, is no hitting others and no banging on the floor with the instruments. If this were to happen, the instrument would have to go back into the music basket to rest!

I step and step and step and step, and then I turn around,
I step and step and step and step then stop without a sound;
I play down low and I play up high;
I play to the earth and I play to the sky;
I step and step and step and step; and then I sit right down.

Baby Hippo's New Teeth

The idea for this story poem came from a group workshop in Nairobi in response to a need for a creative strategy for a three-year-old girl who was always biting others whenever she was upset. It has been written with lots of repetition and rhyme to suit the attention span of this young age group. It was suggested at the workshop that the story could be presented to the child, or to a group of young children, as a simple puppet show (using the child's toys as the puppets).

In China the story has been used by teachers and parents and changed to 'Baby Panda's New Teeth' with animals like 'little squirrel' and 'little monkey' used as friends … but keeping the tortoise in the last section of the story.

Baby Hippo had new teeth,
But she wasn't sure how to use them.
Baby Hippo liked new friends
But she seemed to always lose them!

When little zebra came to play,
Baby Hippo bit her friend,
So little zebra wouldn't stay.
Little zebra went away.

When little giraffe came to play,
Baby Hippo bit her friend,
So little giraffe wouldn't stay.
Little giraffe went away.

When little baboon came to play,
Baby Hippo bit her friend,
So little baboon wouldn't stay.
Little baboon went away.

Then one day,
Little tortoise came to play.
Baby Hippo bit her friend,
But OUCH – Tortoise's back was hard and strong,
OUCH – Baby Hippo didn't bite tortoise for too long!

Wise little tortoise stayed to play,
And showed Baby Hippo a new way.
'Come and bite the grass so sweet,
Grass is good for hippos to eat.'

So Baby Hippo used her teeth,
To bite and chew the grass so sweet.
When her friends would come to play,
The friends would stay and play all day!

The Party in the Jungle

This idea came from a group workshop in Nairobi in response to a need for a story for a six-year-old girl who was always throwing things.

Once upon a time, all the animal friends in the jungle decided to hold a party. They wanted to come together and make music. Each animal had to bring an instrument.

The zebra brought some black-and-white-striped rhythm sticks.
The impala brought a thin brown flute.
The elephant brought a long grey trumpet.
The buffalo brought a fat white horn.

The monkey wanted to come to the party but he couldn't think of any instrument to play, so he decided to have some fun in a different way. He climbed high up in the palm trees above the party.

Up in my tree a zebra I see, if I throw a coconut what fun it could be.

Each time the monkey would say this, he would throw down a coconut to try to hit one of the animals playing music.

Up in my tree an impala I see, if I throw a coconut what fun it could be.
Up in my tree an elephant I see, if I throw a coconut what fun it could be.
Up in my tree a buffalo I see, if I throw a coconut what fun it could be.

The animals didn't like the game the monkey was playing, but they didn't know what to do.

Then the tall giraffe had an idea. He very quietly reached up through the palm leaves and, using his long giraffe tongue, he lifted the monkey out of his hiding place. The giraffe was planning to carry him down to the river and drop him in the water.

But the quick-thinking monkey, who was still holding a coconut tightly in his hands, started to play it like a drum, singing loudly as he played,

In my hands a coconut I play, if I play it like a drum, then please can I stay?

Of course the animals were delighted to have a drummer join their party! So the monkey was invited to stay and play his coconut like a drum. And together all the animal friends had lots of musical fun.

The Stick that Sings

A poem (or story 'seed') for children 'stuck' in gun play, and for children who like to use sticks in hurting or aggressive ways. This idea could be used to encourage positive use of sticks for children aged three to eight.

A child is playing outside and a small stick falls from a tree and lands in front of the child. It is long and smooth and straight. The child picks it up and the stick sings to it – it is a magic stick and here is its song!

I am your new friend, a magic stick,
With your help I can work many tricks,
There are more like me, lying under trees.
Look around – you'll be surprised what you see!

Many long ones of me can build a tee-pee,
Use small ones for houses for garden pixies.
Make long roads or fences – what else can you try?
Two crossed sticks can start a woven god's–eye.

Use me for digging holes in the sand,
And drawing pictures, what fun for your hands.
Jump over many of me laid out on the ground,
Or hold one stick to roll a big ball around.

For catching fish, I can hold a strong line,
Make a flag for my end, or a banner fine,
Two of us can make music, in rhythm we clap,
Or bang on a drum, rap-a-tap-tap.

With a sock on my end I turn into a horse,
You can ride me inside (not too fast of course!).
You can ride me outside, have adventures all day,
Lets go – over hills and away, faraway!

Little Roo

The idea for this story came from a group workshop in Singapore in response to a need for a strategy for a four-year-old boy who was continually hitting other children.

In a land far, far away, there lived two friends, Little Roo and Little Dingo.

These friends used to meet at the waterhole when their families came down to drink water each day. They loved to do things together – slide down the muddy bank, splash in the water, and play hide-and-seek amongst the willow trees growing by the edge of the waterhole.

But as Little Roo grew bigger and stronger, he began to use his kangaroo hands to punch his friend. Little Roo thought this was such fun, he would even sing while he punched:

Punching, punching, all the day, I love to punch so much this way.

Little Dingo didn't think this new game was any fun at all, and tried to avoid going near his friend. Little Roo would chase Little Dingo, singing out:

Punching, punching, all the day, I love to punch so much this way.

Finally Little Dingo's family found another waterhole to visit each day, and Little Roo was left all alone at his waterhole with no one to play with. He tried to punch the tree instead, singing out:

Punching, punching, all the day, I love to punch so much this way.

But the wooden trunk of the old willow tree was too hard for his hands. OUCH – this hurt! Little Kangaroo gave up playing this kind of game. Little Roo didn't like getting hurt.

Time passed, and the rainy season came. While the rains were falling Little Roo's family didn't bother to visit the waterhole as they could find water to drink everywhere and anywhere across the land – in little pools in the rocks and in little streams flowing through the long grasses.

Finally the rains stopped, the land dried out, and Little Roo's family returned to the waterhole to drink. But things looked quite different – the rain had washed some of the new baby willow trees down the muddy bank and into the water, and old Mother Willow was crying out for help.

Little Roo used his strong hands to pick up the baby trees, one by one, and carry them further up the bank, away from the slippery muddy edge. He then dug some holes in the rich brown earth, and planted the baby willows into new and safe homes.

It felt so good to use his hands in this way. Suddenly his hands didn't feel like punching any more, but felt happy and content, like never before.

From this time on, Mother Willow and all her baby trees became Little Roo's new friends. They invited Little Roo and his family to sleep under their shade through the hot summer days.

As the smaller waterholes dried up, Little Dingo and his family returned to Little Roo's waterhole, and they shared the shade of the willow trees through the long hot summer.

Little Roo and Little Dingo were happy to be back together again. They slid down the muddy bank, splashed in the water, and played in the shade of the new willow trees. When the wind blew strongly, the willow branches bent down and tickled their backs, and the willow leaves sang rustling songs to help them sleep.

Buddy Cuddle
by Alfira Fisher

Buddy Cuddle was written at a Creative Discipline workshop in Murwillumbah, NSW, for a brother and sister (aged three and four). They loved the story instantly. It made them laugh and they asked to hear it over and over again. They loved being silly with words and this humour was one of the best ways to lighten difficult and challenging interactions between them. It contains the seed to search for a loving solution. Children can be encouraged to use the words and movement of 'stamp the ground and turn around' to redirect or transform negative into positive behaviour.

Once upon a time there was a little boy and little girl who lived in a home with their Mummy and Daddy, near where the mountains catch the clouds in the sky. The boy and girl were very close, and usually played well together.

One day however, while they were in a cross mood with each other, a mischievous fairy, who liked to cast magic spells on people, turned them both into two different children, called Grump and Grumbellina. After a very grumbly time together, they were both feeling tired and fed up. So they went to see their friend Buddy Cuddle, hoping he could help them get rid of the grumbly spell.

Buddy Cuddle lived in their back garden, in a very cute house, painted all the colours of the rainbow, with a knocking door that would only open with a magic rhyme.

Grump and Grumbellina knew exactly what to say:

Oh what a muddle
Fuddy Muddy Bubble
Come on out to play
Mister Buddy Cuddle.

The door opened and Buddy Cuddle jumped with joy to see his two friends. He gave them a big Huggle Puggle.

The two children told him all about their grumbly day. So he taught them some magic words to get rid of the grumbly spell:

Huff puff, gruff and stuff
Stomp the ground and turn around
Huff puff, gruff and stuff.

They said the magic words together, stomping and turning around

Huff puff, gruff and stuff
Stomp the ground and turn around
Huff puff, gruff and stuff.

Huff puff, gruff and stuff
Stomp the ground and turn around
Huff puff, gruff and stuff.

After this, the grumbles were gone and they had a fun time playing together with Buddy Cuddle until it was time to go home for supper.

The Sailor Boy

The idea for this story came from a primary teachers' training module in Nairobi. It arose in response to the need for a strategy for an eight-year-old child who was damaging things in the classroom and around the school compound. The child's tribal group was from western Kenya and the child had spent his early years on the shores of Lake Victoria – hence was very familiar with fishing.

There was once a fisher family who lived on the shores of a great lake. Every day the father would go out fishing while the mother stayed home and took care of the house and garden. There was only one child in this family, a young boy.

For many years the boy had been happy to stay home with his mother, playing in the garden and on the beach. The young boy had now reached an age where he thought he was old enough to go with his father out on the lake to fish, but his father had told him he must wait a few more years.

Every day the boy watched his father go fishing without him, and every day the boy grew more and more angry about being left behind. One night, when his parents were asleep, the boy crept down to the beach and, in the shining light of the moon, he started to damage things in his father's boat. Firstly he tangled up the fishing line, and then he found his father's fishing knife. 'Oh, ho,' he thought to himself, 'I can have some fun with this.' He set to work angrily digging into his father's water bottle, making holes everywhere and watching the water spurt out all over the bottom of the boat. Then he stabbed the knife into the wooden paddle, making cuts all over the handle, and doing his best to break the blade.

While the young boy was busy with his cutting and stabbing, a strong wind blew up and washed a giant wave up the beach. The wave picked up the boat with the boy inside and carried it back out onto the lake. The boy was helpless to do anything, and ended up falling asleep in the bottom of the boat while waves crashed all around him.

The next day dawned clear and bright. The wind had stopped and the sun was shining. The young boy woke up and looked out to see the shoreline far in the distance. He was very thirsty, but the water bottle was empty so he had nothing to drink. He was also hungry, and thought, 'perhaps I could catch a fish'. But there were so many knots in the fishing line it was impossible to use it. Then the boy tried to use the paddle to row the boat ashore, but the handle of the paddle had so many knife cuts in it that it soon snapped in half. What use is half a paddle when you are many miles from shore?

Then the boy looked into the bottom of the boat and noticed the knife he had tried to break the night before. He picked it up and was relieved to see that the blade was bent but not broken. The giant wave must have washed him out to sea before he could do that kind of damage!

With the tip of the knife he found he could get into the knots of the fishing line and he slowly began to unravel the tangles. Soon he was able to use a long length of line to tie around the broken paddle and make it strong again.

With the mended paddle in his hands, he began the long journey back home. As he came closer to the shoreline, he could see his father and mother waiting on the beach. His father swam out to meet him then dragged the boat back to shallow water. His mother picked him up and carried him to the house, and dressed him in warm, dry clothes. She then fed him a large pot of warm porridge and some hot tea, and tucked him into bed. Both his parents seemed so happy to have him alive and safely home.

And how happy he was to be alive and safely home! The previous night now just seemed like a bad dream, and soon, with his mother singing lullabies to him, he fell into a deep and comfortable sleep.

The Scratchy Spiky Porcupine

The idea for this story came from a group workshop in Singapore. The teachers at the WCNC Daycare Centre wanted a creative strategy for a three-and-a-half-year-old child who was scratching other children. The parents didn't want to cut the child's nails (a practical strategy for this situation), so the teachers worked successfully with a story to help the child use her hands in careful ways.

Once upon a time, Porcupine and her friends were going on a walk through the forest. It was a beautiful day and they had decided to go to the river to have a picnic.

Porcupine pushed past each of her friends as they walked along. Porcupine wanted to be first to the river. Porcupine always wanted to be first whenever she went anywhere with her friends. But she didn't realize that her sharp spikes scratched each of her friends as she pushed past them.

Once Porcupine was in the lead she ran ahead and disappeared along the path. When she reached the river she turned around to look for her friends, but they were nowhere to be seen. Porcupine walked back through the forest, looking to one side of the path and then the other. Finally she found them, busy in the bushes, gathering thick shiny leaves.

'What are you doing?' she asked her friends.

'We are making you a special coat,' answered her friends, 'so your sharp quills can't scratch us anymore.'

The friends put the thick leaves over Porcupine's body until all her sharp quills were covered with a soft coat of shiny green.

Then the friends walked happily to the river and sat on the riverbank and enjoyed a picnic together.

The Wandering Gnome with the Kind Hands
by Dawn Tranter

Note from the author: A five-year-old boy in my kindergarten would pinch or hit other children regularly but always without being observed. Initially I worked with rubbing 'kind hand-cream' into his hands but not with great success, and so I wrote this story. With the storytelling each day, a different child would have a turn to be the gnome. I had a beautiful crystal bowl filled with water and this gnome would have his hands washed with the waters from the 'well of kindness'. One day this particular child asked if he could be the gnome. By coincidence he had been climbing a pine tree and had sticky brown colour on his hands – which were then washed clean! After this story (I told it daily for two weeks) the pinching and hitting ceased.

Once upon a time, in a land far away, there lived a troop of gnomes ruled by a king who was strong and firm, but also kind. These hardworking gnomes were strong and healthy, and worked for their king with pleasure.

Mornings would find this little troop of gnomes tickling the roots of the plant children to waken them. Later in the day they would dig in the earth searching for crystals for their king. At the end of a hard day's work, the king always made sure the gnomes had good, nourishing food to eat, and he always spoke words of kindness, thanking them for their hard work and loyalty.

All was well in this kingdom, until one day a little gnome from another kingdom came to stay. At first he was made welcome, for he too seemed hard-working and kind. But as the days went on this little gnome became more and more unkind. When it was time to awaken the plant children, instead of tickling their roots he would pull, quite hard, hurting the plant children dreadfully. When the little troop went off to dig for crystals, he would follow behind, and when no one was looking, he would push the little gnome in front of him, making him fall and hurt himself. After the good gnomes had dug their crystals up, he would take them, not wanting to do the hard work for himself.

At last the kind gnomes had endured enough, and decided they would have nothing more to do with this unkind gnome.

At the same time that the kind gnomes wanted nothing more to do with him, this little gnome began to notice something very odd, something very awful … his hands were changing, and becoming hard! Every time he pulled a plant in a hurting way, his soft hands became harder; every time he squashed a beetle his hands grew stiffer and harder; every time he pushed one of his friends, his hands became stiffer and harder. They were even changing to a terrible colour! With every passing day, his hands were becoming worse. At last he went to the king, and said: 'What is happening, what is happening, make it stop, please can you help me?'

The old king in his wisdom sat in silence for a time, then said, 'Yes, I can help you, but before I give you something to do that could help, you must promise that from this day forth you will use your hands to be helpful and kind. You must promise that all your deeds will be done with good kind hands'. 'I promise, I promise', said the little gnome, 'what must I do?'

The old king told him, 'Every day you must visit the well deep inside the mountain. By the well sits an old woman; you must ask her to bathe your hands in the waters from the well of kindness. You must ask her to bathe your hands every day until you feel them begin to soften, until you feel the goodness and kindness in your hands.'

And so, every day, this little gnome went to the well deep in the mountain, and every day the old woman, with great patience and great gentleness, bathed the hands of the little gnome, singing all the while,

With hands so soft and hands so kind, with gentleness for all of time.

Day after day the little gnome's hands were bathed, and day after day the old woman sang,

With hands so soft and hands so kind, with gentleness for all of time.

At first the little gnome thought it all a waste of time: his hands were still hard and quite a dreadful colour. But as time went on the little gnome began to feel his hands changing; at first it was hardly noticeable, but then the hardness went, and the colour changed. The little gnome could feel the goodness and kindness coming into his hands, he could really feel it!

Finally there came a day when the old woman of the well bathed the little gnome's hands for the last time. She dried his gentle hands with great reverence and held them in her kind, old hands, then bid the little gnome farewell.

The little gnome went straight back to the king and thanked him most sincerely for his help. 'You are very welcome', said the king, 'and now you must go out and fulfil your promise to use your hands only for good, kind deeds.'

And do you know, that is just what the little gnome did! He travelled from kingdom to kingdom, offering assistance wherever and whenever he could help. And everywhere he went, people always spoke of the wandering gnome with the kind, kind hands.

The Red Berries and the Handy Squirrel
by Laura Hurtado-Roberts

This story idea came out of a therapeutic storytelling workshop in Wellington, New Zealand. Note by Laura: This story is based on my experience of helping an autistic child with whom I worked for eight months in New Zealand. He was 10 at the time but equivalent to 6–7 years because of his development delay. The main factor was that when I was using bean bags to help his hands in throwing or catching, or just passing them around the body doing different movements, he could not do these at all. His hands and fingers were only forming signs learned for expressing 'bad words' and he was distracted by this. After several lessons his mother was embarrassed by what he was doing, and asked me if I could stop these exercises. This was the reason I wrote the story! I used the story twice in my sessions when I gave him a footbath and massage, so he was calm and listened carefully to it. After hearing the story several times he came back with a page on which he had written his thoughts about many positive uses of his hands: 'I use my hands for giving, for clapping' … After this, the negative behaviour changed!

The story had helped the boy to love his hands and see the positive things that he could do with them. Also, in his next drawing, he drew a person with hands! (Before this, his drawings were of people without hands.) The boy loved the story and kept it with him. His mum was also very grateful.

Once upon a time there was a mummy bird with a little yellow baby bird. They lived in a basket-shaped nest woven by twigs and leaves and softened with feathers. Their cosy home was on the top branch of a high oak tree. They were happily living together in their nest, and the yellow birdie was learning how to feed himself, and how to fly. The days passed and he was keen to get out of the nest and go to explore the forest. One day mummy bird said to him: 'There will be no more food left in a couple of days and winter is getting closer. I must go out and bring some food but it will take me some days to get back. So you may explore close to home but do not go into that dark bush over there' – and she pointed with her beak toward the west – 'because that bush is very thick and it is not safe to go there on your own.'

But the yellow birdie was busy preening himself, and could not see where the deep dark bush was. Nevertheless he was proud of gaining his independence. The bright sunshine encouraged him to explore, and forage, and happily fly over the forest. He found a stream where he could get some water, and saw some worms in the mud. But he said, *I must look further around*, and he started flying higher and higher, so high in his excitement that he flew around in circles in the sky. Then suddenly he realized that he had forgotten how to find his way home.

Despite the dazzling sunlight he could just make out some red berries and his mouth was watering at the thought of his first feast of berries. The light was so strong that he could not see that the bush was the dark and deep bush that mother bird had said not to go into. With excited movements, the little fledgling tried to get as many berries as he could, but a huge net tangled his feet and wings and he thrashed about in the net but was unable to get out. He fell silent and was frightened, and the image of his mum came to him, with her words: 'Don't go into that dark bush … ' Well, it was too late: the only thing to do was to sing and call for help.

His sound was sharp and he sang many times expecting that perhaps his mother was around and would hear him. However, next to the berry bush there were a few walnut trees where some squirrels were gathering nuts because winter was just around the corner. One of the squirrels heard the bird's song and decided to see what was happening. He climbed and jumped through some trees and got closer to the berry bush, where he saw a bird tangled in a net. He said: 'Don't be afraid, I can help you, I have strong hands and with my paws I can untangle the net. How did you get trapped in there?'

Birdie said that it was his first outing and he had been attracted by the red colour of the berries. The sunshine was so dazzling that he could not see the net. 'Well,' the squirrel said, 'trust your new friend, in a couple of minutes you will be free.' Then the squirrel added: 'It is nearly night, wait until the sun comes up tomorrow morning before you go back home. There are some holes in the walnut trees where you can sleep peacefully.' Birdie smiled and his heart was cheerful and confident again. He had made a new friend, who had helpful and friendly hands.

Helpful hands can do a lot of things!
If I move my fingers gently and kindly I can feel different textures, such as my mum's softness, or I can give a friendly pat on my brother's shoulder. If I want to do useful things with my hands, I can help my mum to do things with tools, like a hammer, or I can even knead bread with my palms.
Yes, my hands, like the squirrel's paws, are my friends.
With them I can give and receive lovely gifts and help.
My hands are my friends!

Little Lead Pencil
by Melanie Turner

Note from Melanie: Hi Susan. I came to your workshop in Moruya. We spoke about my son Pippin (age five) who had been labelled a 'scribbler' by his teacher and had broken pencils in defiance. I wrote the attached story to give to his teacher to read to the class. When my husband read it, I explained that the boy in the story was actually a metaphor for the teacher and the pencil was the metaphor for our son, and a tear came to his eye – he remembered having the same experience at school of having his work thrown in the bin for not being good enough!

I gave the story to Pippin's teacher to read to the class. I asked her not to let my son know that I had written it, so that he wouldn't know it was about him. The next day, while I was helping Pippin do his homework, he commented on his work 'Mummy, I just made a beautiful "a". I said, 'That's good, it looks like you and your pencil are becoming friends'. He then told me about a story that the teacher had read at school about a boy and his pencil and he told me about the song and tried to remember the verse. I said 'Oh that sounds like a good story; I might have to get a copy so that we can read it at home.' I then told Pippin's other teacher about the story and the positive result and she asked for a copy; and another teacher who was listening also requested a copy to use for her year 2 students. I'm

*so proud of myself! It was so much fun to work like this, 'behind the scenes'
… very inspiring and satisfying.*

Once there was a Little Lead Pencil who lived in the kindergarten
classroom. Little Lead Pencil loved living in the kindergarten classroom because the teacher was always reading stories, and listening to
stories was Little Lead Pencil's favourite thing to do.

Little Lead Pencil dreamed of one day writing a story of its own,
a wonderful tale of adventure and mystery just like the stories that it
loved to hear.

The day came when the kindergarten children were learning to
write the letters of the alphabet. Little Lead Pencil was really excited
because it knew that this was the first step in learning to write stories.
All the pencils in the tin were paired up with a child in the class ready
for the lesson. Little Lead Pencil was paired with a boy who was just
learning to write. This boy was a very fast learner who had already
learnt to read, in fact he was used to doing everything very quickly,
but what the boy didn't know was that learning to write letters can
take a lot of time and practice.

The boy picked up the Little Lead Pencil and held it very tightly
in his hand. He quickly finished the worksheet as fast as he could.
But when the teacher came to check the children's work, all she could
see from Little Lead Pencil were scribbles. The boy had pushed the
pencil so hard and fast around the page that scribbles were all Little
Lead Pencil could make.

So the boy had to start the worksheet again. He became very angry
with Little Lead Pencil. Because he had to do the worksheet again, he
wouldn't be the first to finish in the class, which meant he couldn't be the
first to go on to the next activity. 'This time,' thought the boy, 'I will have
to push this pencil really hard to make it go where I want it to go.' He
grabbed Little Lead Pencil and pushed it hard on the page, but Little Lead
Pencil did not like being pushed and grabbed and it only made scribbles
on the page, so the boy pushed harder still and faster and harder until
Little Lead Pencil could not take any more and broke into two pieces.

The teacher was not pleased! When the children were at lunch she
took the broken pieces of Little Lead Pencil. There was still a piece
of pencil that would be ok, so she sharpened this piece to make a
smaller pencil and she put the smaller pencil back in the pencil tin.

That night when the children were all at home in their beds, Little
Lead Pencil was very sad. All it wanted was to write a story of its own, full
of adventure and mystery. What could it do, how could it make the boy

understand that he needed to guide the pencil gently, without squeezing or pushing too hard? How could it let the boy know that it needed more time to glide along the page in order to make beautiful letters?

Little Lead Pencil came up with a plan. It jumped out of the pencil tin and onto a spare piece of paper and in its most beautiful and best writing it wrote this song:

> *Hold me gently in your hand*
> *Then softly on the page I'll land*
> *Guide me gently on the page*
> *Watch me dancing, like on stage*
> *Lead me slowly, gently round*
> *Watch me dance, without a sound*
> *Circles round and lines so straight*
> *Lovely letters you will make.*

The next morning, when the children came into the class, there, sitting on the boy's desk was a piece of paper with a song on it, the one that Little Lead Pencil had written. The boy read the song and at once knew the message had come from Little Lead Pencil. The words on the note were written so neatly and beautifully that the boy took the note and put it in his bag, for he wanted to take it home and hang it up so that he could always look at it. And when the time came to practise writing, the boy knew exactly what to do.

It took time for the boy to learn how to hold Little Lead Pencil as in the song, but because he was being gentler with Little Lead Pencil and giving it more time, they soon became great friends. The boy would sing the song softly to himself when he needed help with writing letters. With Little Lead Pencil's help the boy was able to write beautiful and neat letters, just like in the song. Eventually the boy and Little Lead Pencil wrote a wonderful tale of adventure and mystery ... but that's another story!

The Elephant's Trunk

The idea for this story came out of a workshop in Sydney. It was in response to the need for a creative strategy for a five-year-old boy who was continually using his hands to hurt others. The elephant was this boy's favourite animal. The story could be best told as a puppet show using some toy elephants to give the visual effect of the 'rescue' – a rope made from trunks and tails!

Note: The main character could be changed to a monkey and the story could be based around a monkey family – this would also work well with a rescue 'rope' made from monkeys' hands and monkeys' tails.

There was once a young elephant called Tembo. Tembo was one of the strongest young elephants in the herd. But he was always using his strong trunk to bash and thrash things. He would bash and thrash the trees, and bash and thrash any small animals he met on the path. His brothers and sisters tried to stay clear of him as he bashed and thrashed his way through the day. Even the ox-pecker birds that landed on the backs of the elephants in the herd, stayed clear of Tembo. They couldn't trust what he might do with his strong trunk.

As Tembo went about his hurting business, he would shout out for all to hear him:

> *Bash and thrash, bash and thrash, my trunk is so strong – I can bash and thrash.*

Old Grandmother Elephant kept warning Tembo to be more careful. 'Your trunk should be a helping trunk, not a hurting trunk,' she would say to her young and reckless grandson.

But Tembo didn't take any notice of Grandmother Elephant. He just kept on bashing and thrashing things, shouting as he went along with the herd:

> *Bash and thrash, bash and thrash, my trunk is so strong – I can bash and thrash.*

One day, on their journey to find a new source of water, the elephant herd reached a rocky ravine. Grandmother Elephant led the way, slowly and carefully, across a waterfall and along the edge of a steep, rocky cliff. Tembo and the other young elephants followed her, but Tembo was so busy trying to bash into one of his brothers that he tripped and fell at the top of the waterfall. Down, down, down he went, sliding on his elephant bottom over the wet rocks – all the way down to splash into a pool of water far below.

Tembo was frightened to be at the bottom of the waterfall all by himself. He bashed and thrashed around the edges, trying to get out, but the rocks were too slippery. No matter how loud he sang his song, it didn't seem to be of any help:

> *Bash and thrash, bash and thrash, my trunk is so strong – I can bash and thrash.*

Meanwhile, at the top of the cliffs, Grandmother Elephant had come to the rescue. She was using her trunk in a very strong way. Her trunk was curling tightly around Tembo's brother's tail and it was slowly lowering him down the rocky cliff. When his brother reached the edge of the pool, he stretched out his little trunk to take hold of Tembo's tail. Slowly, slowly, Tembo found himself being pulled backwards out of the pool. Slowly, slowly, backwards up the rocky cliff.

Slowly, slowly, Tembo was pulled by Grandmother's long and strong trunk, and his brother's small but strong trunk – all the way to safety. The elephants' trunks and tails had made a rescue rope. Tembo could not believe what had happened!

From that day onwards, Tembo understood a different way to use his strong trunk. And he used a different song as he walked along:

Lift and carry, hold and pull, my trunk is so strong –
I can lift and carry, hold and pull, all day long!

With his new song, and a new way to make use of his strong trunk, Tembo now found many things to do – he could reach up high and pull juicy branches down to eat, he could lift big logs out of the path to make it easier for the new baby elephants to follow their mothers, and when he was down at the river he could pick up the water and spray it all over his back to cool himself down.

And sometimes, just for fun, Tembo and his brothers and sisters would link tails and trunks, and walk the elephant paths in a long single line.

If you go travelling in the African bush, and you see elephants using their trunks like this, it might be Tembo using his strong trunk, walking in a long line with his family.

'Story bones' – knights, dragons and princesses

The Knights and the Dragon

This story idea was created at a workshop in Hobart for a ten-year-old boy who was always losing his temper and throwing/destroying things. The 'bones' of the story are presented here for you to work with – these 'bones' are quite substantial and could be the basis for a 'quest' story or even a book of several chapters.

Two strong knights set off on a journey but along the way are continually arguing about who is the best – they have a sword-throwing contest to see who can throw the furthest (and both swords get lost); they have a horse-racing contest (both horses set off on a race and don't return); they have a shield-breaking contest (drop large rocks off a cliff onto the shields and both get broken).

The two knights are left sword-less, horseless, and shield-less – they come to a river, bend down to get a drink, and both see in their reflection a dragon standing behind them, but when they stand up and look around the dragon is gone (note: the dragon is a symbol of their fiery anger and it only lives in the reflection).

The knights begin the long journey back home – on the way they have to find food and shelter – one gets a sore leg and the other helps him walk, one gets sick and the other finds herbs to make him better – eventually they get back to their king's castle – as they are crossing the castle moat, they stop on the bridge and look into the water – the dragon is no longer there in the reflection.

The Princess and the River

This story idea was created at a workshop in Nairobi for a five-year-old girl who was continually hitting her brothers and sisters. The 'bones' of the story are presented here for you to flesh out into a full story.

Story about a princess who lived near a river and wanted to find a way to cross over – her younger sister princess lived on the other side and would wave to her and call out to her to come over and play – but the river was quite deep and wild – princess tried to ride her horse across, horse not so happy about being in the wild river and the princess would get so cross and hit the horse and the horse would rear up and refuse to move – many times the princess would get onto her horse and try to cross over, and many times the horse would not make it across. Finally a wise monkey told the princess to look down in the water as she was riding her horse and this would show her the way to go – 'Little Princess as you're going, look down to see what the river's showing' – the princess took the wise monkey's advice, climbed onto the horse's back and as they stepped in the river she looked down. She was surprised to see her hands hitting out at the horse – so this time she used her hands to hold the reins and pat the horse and slowly she guided it all the way across. When she reached the other side she spent the whole day having a wonderful time with her sister princess. From this time on the two princesses were able to play together every day, as the older sister had learnt how to cross the deep and wild river by herself.

4

Anxious/Insecure/Fearful

The Shadow Giant

'Greed is my game and Power is my name' … a story for children at a time of floods, bush fires, tsunamis, earthquakes and man-made disasters.

My work with therapeutic story-writing has taken me to many countries over the years, and as I travel I encounter more and more requests for therapeutic stories for our 'global crisis' situation, from peoples in Africa to Asia to the UK and the US. This story was written in the wake of the earthquakes in Haiti and New Zealand, the oil spill in the Gulf of Mexico, the floods and bushfires in Australia, the tsunami and nuclear disaster in Japan and the growing concern over chemical pollution and food shortages, especially in developing countries. My aim is to reach primary- and high-school children in an imaginative way to encourage discussion and debate. An Australian environmentalist described the story message as 'simple but poignant'.

Once upon a time, in the not-so-distant past, there lived a giant who was the strongest, largest and most destructive creature ever to have lived on earth.

The mysterious thing was that no one had ever seen the giant, but many had experienced its dark shadow as it travelled around the earth, leaving destruction in it wake. People called it the Shadow Giant.

The Shadow Giant was continually busy, day and night, night and day, moving around the world, stamping its dark presence on the earth, in the ocean and in the air … deep black cracks in the ground, engulfing waves of black water and mud on the coastlines, burnt and blackened forests in the valleys and the mountains, and swirling masses of polluting fog everywhere.

No one knew where the Shadow Giant came from and where it lived. And no one knew when and where it would next use its dark force.

Nothing was safe from this giant – not the peoples of the world, nor the animals of the land, nor the creatures of the sea. All were vulnerable to its power. Even the birds, who could usually fly fast enough to escape its path of destruction, were slowly being affected by the swirling black fog spreading through the air.

The Queen of the Heavens, who lived high up in her Silver Castle above the clouds, heard news of these terrible events from her feathered messengers, the birds. She was growing ever more concerned about the Shadow Giant and the evil work it was doing on the earth below. She decided to call a meeting and sent out an invitation to all the birds of the air, everywhere in the world.

On the day of the meeting, the Queen of the Heavens was seated on her silver throne, resplendent in her flowing rainbow gown. All around her were gathered many birds: birds from every part of the world, birds of all colours and shapes and sizes, birds of the land and birds of the sea, birds of the day and birds of the night.

Patiently and intently the Queen of the Heavens listened to each and every bird – between them they had seen every kind of destruction caused by the Shadow Giant. When all the stories had been told, the Queen spoke to the gathering:

'There must be a way to overcome this dark force that is taking over the earth. Every enemy has a weakness! Fly back where you have come from and try to find where the Shadow Giant lives – then you can observe what weakness it may have. Report back to me as soon as you can … There is not a moment to lose!'

So the birds flew back to their homes around the world and kept a vigilant watch on the giant's path of destruction, trying to track down where it lived. Days passed, weeks passed, months passed.

When it was almost a year since the birds had been sent on their quest, an old owl finally found the answer the Queen was looking for. He was flying into a deep mountain cave, searching for something to eat, and he followed a tunnel which led into a large rock cavern.

Inside this cavern was a huge, dark, mumbling, rumbling figure. It was of no definite shape, in fact its shape seemed to change size and form with every sound it made. Sometimes it filled most of the cavern like a giant squid with many writhing tentacles, other times it turned into a monstrous bear-like figure and stamped angrily around the cave

The owl hid in a far corner of the cavern and watched and listened, as owls can do very well. After a while he began to make some sense of the repeatedly chanted mumblings and rumblings:

All for me and me for all, devouring all things big and small,
Greed is my game and Power is my name.

Finally the hideous dark creature curled itself into a large ball and fell asleep. The owl quickly and quietly flew out of the deep mountain cave. Then he began the long journey across the sky, all the way to the castle of the Queen of the Heavens. As he flew higher and higher, he kept chanting the awful mumbling rumblings so he would not forget them.

All for me and me for all, devouring all things big and small,
Greed is my game and Power is my name.

When the Queen of the Heavens heard the story from the owl, she had no doubt that he had found the home of the Shadow Giant. And when she heard the mumbling rumbling chant, she immediately recognized the Giant's weakness: *The Shadow Giant only cares for itself – it only wants power for itself!'*

Then the Queen of the Heavens called for her feathered helpers. 'Fly out around the world and sing this message to the people. If they work together and care for each other then they can slowly but surely overcome this dark shadow that is harming the earth.'

Strength in caring, strength in togetherness, can overcome the giant's
selfishness.

The birds flew out to all parts of the world, birds of all colours and shapes and sizes, birds of the land and birds of the sea, birds of the day and birds of the night. And as they flew, they sang the message from the Queen of the Heavens for all on earth to hear.

And to this day, the birds are still singing their song. Sometimes they even drop feather messages which flutter softly to the ground. When the people find these beautiful feathers lying on the ground … in the garden, on the street, in the forest and on the beach … they know that this message has been sent directly to them. They pick up the feathers, they wonder at their form and beauty, and they remember the message that has been sent to them by the Queen of the Heavens.

Strength in caring, strength in togetherness!

And slowly but surely, the wisdom of the song of the birds is helping the people of the world to overcome the dark power of the Shadow Giant.

The Rose and the Thorn

A story for the Children of Norway, written by Susan Perrow with help from Eldbjorg and Dieter Paulsen, Arendal, Norway (see Chapter One (page 23) for background context).

There was once a prince and a princess who lived in a castle surrounded by a beautiful garden. In this garden grew many kinds of flowers, but the most beautiful of all was the rose bush. This rose bush was like no other – it had one perfect red rose that never seemed to grow old. And it had a smooth green stem and smooth green branches without any thorns.

People came from far and wide to look at such perfection … a rose without thorns that never seemed to die! Every day the prince and princess would walk through their garden and stop to give thanks for the wonder and beauty of this rose.

However, deep in the rose bush, hiding far down inside the stem, there was a long sharp thorn that was bursting to find its way out. It had been living in the rose bush for a very long time and slowly, slowly, slowly, it was making its way upwards. As it travelled up through the green stem it knocked against the woody edges but these were too strong for the thorn to push through.

Then one day the long sharp thorn reached the top of the bush, where the soft red rose sat shining in the sun. Here was an easy doorway for the long sharp thorn! It pierced right through the heart of the red rose and came out into the daylight.

As the thorn broke through the heart of the rose, all the red petals fell off and fluttered to the ground. When the prince and princess were walking in their garden later that day they were shocked at what they found. Their beautiful red rose had died, all its petals had been blown across the garden and the stem and branches were withered and brown. The only thing left shining in the late afternoon light was one silver thorn, pointing high to the sky.

The prince and princess quickly called for the castle gardeners to come and dig out the dead rose bush. Then they returned to the castle to mourn the loss of the beautiful red rose. That night a heavy fog settled upon the gardens.

However, the next morning the fog had disappeared, and the day dawned clear and bright. When the prince and princess looked out of their castle window a most wondrous sight met their eyes. Wherever a rose petal had landed in the garden, a rose bush had taken root, had grown tall and strong and was budding with new rose flowers.

As the sun climbed across the sky, each of the new rose buds opened their petals to the light. There were many different roses of many different perfumes and many different colours – yellow, orange, blue, purple, pink, red and white. The prince and princess walked out into the garden with joy and hope in their hearts, and people came from far and wide to give thanks for the wonder and beauty of the roses.

The Ants and the Storm

In May 2008 an earthquake measuring 7.8 on the Richter scale hit Chengdu in the heart of Sichuan Province in China. The Chengdu Waldorf School suffered major structural damage, and while thankfully no adult or child in the school community was hurt by the earthquake, the school was closed for many weeks and many families of the school lived in tents in the school ground till repairs could be made to their homes. The kindergarten children were extracted in time from their school building, but watched the walls collapsing and experienced the ground shaking. In a storytelling module in Chengdu I encouraged the teachers to work on the following story to help the very young children understand and cope with the traumatic event. The school has a large pond in the centre of its grounds, and one of the favourite walks for the young children was exploring for insects and birds around the edge of this pond. The teachers used these ideas for their story. They felt that telling it as a simple puppet show, over and over and over again, would help reduce the children's anxiety about the earthquake events.

There was once a large family of ants that lived in many little grass houses near a pond. Around the pond were beautiful willow trees. The ant children played in and out of the fallen willow leaves, and the willow trees shaded the little houses. It was a good place for the ants to live.

One day, however, a big storm came across the valley and blew in the doors and windows of the grass houses. The wind was so strong that even the ground was shaking, and all the ant houses toppled down and fell into cracks in the ground.

Fortunately the mother ants had known of the coming of this big storm. Just in time they led all their children out of their houses and down to the pond. The helping willow trees dropped many leaf boats onto the water, just near the edge of the pond. One by one all the ant families were able to cross onto the leaf boats and stay afloat on the water. The mother ants sang their children to sleep with a soothing lullaby, and they stayed safely on the leaf boats all through the night.

When they woke up the next morning the wind and rain had gone, the ground had stopped shaking and the sun was shining. The leaf boats floated back to the bank and the ants climbed back onto the ground. The mother ants then set to work busily building new houses in the grass.

Soon all was as before. The ant children played in and out of the fallen willow leaves, and the willow trees shaded the new little houses. It was a good place for the ants to live.

The Sparkling River

*I wrote the following story during the devastating floods in Brisbane in January 2011 as a small token of help to the Queensland flood recovery effort. It was used by the Education Department's Teaching and Learning Branch as a resource and put on some blog sites that were established after the flooding. A radio announcer for the ABC Brisbane network talked on air one day of how her six-year-old daughter didn't want to drink water for many months after the floods as she thought 'water was bad' …
I emailed her the story; later she replied that she had shared it with her daughter and 'it had made her day'!*

This story has since been modified and translated into some Filipino languages – Tagalog and Visaya – to be used by teachers in the communities in Southern Philippines which suffer from floods each monsoon season.

There was once a town built on the banks of a long and windy river. The people who lived in the town loved their river – its waters sparkled in the sunshine, many boats moved up and down its lazy flow, bicycles and cars travelled along paths and roads on its banks, and children played in the parks along its banks. By night the moon and stars and the lights of the town were reflected in the river's silky stillness.

The people who lived in the town were proud of their river that sparkled by day and sparkled by night.

At certain times during the year, the rains would fall and the sparkling river would grow brown and swollen and flow swiftly by. But when the rains stopped the river would settle down again, and all would be as clear and sparkling as before.

However, there was a week when the rains fell so heavily that the river filled up and swelled over its banks and into the town. The brown muddy waters flowed into houses and shops and schools. Many people had to move out of their homes and sleep in large halls together, in many beds all in a row.

When the rains stopped the sun shone once again. The brown waters slowly flowed back out of the houses and shops and schools. The brown waters slowly flowed back down the streets and into the river and out into the ocean. As the brown waters flowed back into the river, they left a coating of mud on everything. It took many months and much work for the mud to be cleaned up. It took many months for the river to lose its brown muddy colour and regain its sparkle.

However, during this brown, muddy time, the people of the town discovered a new kind of sparkle. It was a sparkle in the eyes of helping neighbours. It was a sparkle in the eyes of helping strangers. It was a sparkle in the offer of a helping hand that came from all over the land and from faraway lands.

This new kind of sparkle helped give the people of the river town much hope. They carried this with them through all the muddy days and muddy weeks and muddy months.

They carried this with them until once again their river was sparkling in the sunshine.

They carried this with them until once again the moon and stars and the lights of the town were reflected in the river's silky stillness.

The Golden Pipe

This story idea came from discussions at a workshop in Nairobi – it is for a seven-year-old boy who was fearful of going to sleep since his recent school visit to the crocodile farm (before this visit he had never been afraid at night).

There was once a happy boy called Zolo who played in his garden all day long. His favourite place was the large pond filled with golden fish and the boy would spend hours by this pond watching the golden fish swim and dive and jump and dance in the water.

But one day Zolo was surprised and frightened to see that a crocodile had found its way into his pond and frightened all the golden fish away. Zolo immediately ran inside to tell his family what had happened. Zolo's father called in the crocodile catcher and the crocodile was taken back to a deep river far away where it belonged. But from this time onwards, Zolo refused to go outside and the golden fish were not seen again.

One day Zolo's grandfather came to visit and wanted to go with Zolo into the garden but Zolo refused to go outside. Grandfather went out to the pond and pulled out his golden pipe and started to play. While he was playing Zolo was peeping out through the window to watch what was happening. As soon as the golden pipe played beautiful music, the golden fish swam up to the surface of the pond and started to swim and dive and jump and dance in the water.

Zolo ran outside to join his grandfather – he was so happy to see that the golden fish had come back. From that day on, Grandfather taught Zolo how to play the pipe, and Zolo knew he would always have a way to call his golden fish to swim and dive and jump and dance.

The Star Child's Journey

This was a story I wrote in 1986 and used in my preschool ('Periwinkle') in the first few weeks of every new school year. 25 years later, the teachers are still telling it (often as a simple puppet show) as it helps soothe the anxiety of many new children. Parents have often reported that their children came home and told them the story and were keen to return to see the puppet show again and again. Also some parents have used it as a bedtime story to help soothe their child into a 'nightmare'-free sleep. Suitable for age 3–5.

There was once a little Star Child who lived high up in the heavens amongst the stars. His father was Great King Sun and his mother was the Lady of the Moon. All day long he would play with his star brothers and star sisters and he was very happy.

But sometimes little Star Child would look far down into the world below: he could see mountains and rivers and forests and beaches and ocean – so many things to explore. Often he would think, 'How I would love to go on a journey down to the beautiful world below.' But every time he asked his father and mother they would say, 'Not now, little Star Child, you are too young to go on such a journey by yourself.'

One day his father and mother called to him and said, 'Now it is time little Star Child. Now you are old enough to go on this journey. And to help you on your way we have gifts for you.'

His mother, the Lady of the Moon, gave him a soft round moon-boat to journey in by day and to sleep in by night. His father, Great King Sun, gave him a golden sail, made from the rays of the golden sun. 'This sun-sail', said his father, 'will guide your boat through the strongest storms and the darkest nights.'

Little Star Child said goodbye to his father and mother, and climbed into the moon-boat with the golden sun-sail. He then set off on his journey through the starry skies, along the sunbeams, all the way to the blue waters below.

Sail, sail my boat, carry me through starry skies,
Carry me along the sunbeams, sail, sail my boat.

When his boat reached the place where the sky meets the sea, the Dawn Princess was waiting with open arms to lift his boat down and gently set it onto the blue waves.

Sail, sail my boat, carry me across the water, sail, sail my boat.

For many days and nights he journeyed over the water, the sun-sail guiding the way, the moon-boat rocking him to sleep at night, and the Dawn Princess greeting him each new day.

Eventually he came to an island. The little boat landed on a long beach with golden sands, little rock pools and shady green trees.

The Star Child left his little boat to float on a rock pool, and set out walking along the beach. He hadn't walked far when he came across another rock pool. Floating on the water was a large pink and white shell, and playing inside the shell were more little children, just like him.

'Hello' called out the children, 'we are playing in the Periwinkle boat, would you like to come and join us?' So little Star Child climbed inside and had many adventures with his new friends.

The Song of the Seashell

This story was written by Susan Perrow and Phillippa Church for a children's midwinter festival on the east coast of Australia. It captures the natural phenomenon of many whales that pass up the coast each winter on their way north to birth their babies in warmer waters. It could be used with anxious children as a bedtime story for age 4 to 8. It includes a soothing lullaby.

Once upon a time there were many whales living in the coldest part of the world where icy islands float upon the ocean, and where penguins huddle together to keep warm, and sea lions wrap themselves in pelts of fur to keep out the cold blizzards that blow.

Now it happened that the mother whales were growing round and full. They were almost ready to have their babies, but they needed to find warmer waters where their babies could be born, and play together safe and warm. But the whales didn't know how to find their way out of the icy ocean to the warmer waters, so they decided to visit the wise old Sea King and ask for his help.

Down, down, down they swam, deeper than whales usually ever go, all the way down to the deepest, darkest part of the sea, until they came to the Sea King's palace. There they found the Sea King sitting on a throne of seashells, with a crown of pearls in his matted seaweed hair.

'I can help you find your way to the warmer waters' the Sea King said, 'but first I need your help. The great lantern that lights my palace hall is growing very dim, it needs some more golden light. Will you take it to the surface of the ocean where only the whales can go, and fill it with golden sunbeams so it can shine brightly once again, and light up my palace hall through the long dark winter months ahead.'

The whales agreed to the Sea King's request, and they began to pull the great lantern, made from the shell of a giant clam and with windows of finest pearl, up, up, up, to the surface of the ocean, where the water meets the sky. And there, in between the icy islands, they were able to catch the very last of the summer sunbeams that were still dancing with the waves, and put them into the lantern.

With the last of the sunbeams gone, the sea and the sky turned very dark, and only with the golden light of the great lantern were the whales able to find their way back to the Sea King's palace. Down, down, down they swam, pulling the great lantern behind them. The Sea King was very pleased to see them and very pleased to have such a bright golden light in his palace hall once more.

'Now, it is my turn to help you' he said, and he reached down into his treasure chest and lifted out a shining white shell. 'This is a magic seashell and it will lead you wherever you need to go. All you have to do is follow its magic song.'

Then the Sea King let the shell go into the swirling waters outside his palace hall. The shell floated upwards and away. As the whales listened they heard a soft singing

Follow the magic seashell, Listen to its soft song
Leading the whales onwards,
To the place of the warmer waters
Listen to its soft song …

The whales thanked the Sea King and began swimming after the magic seashell, all the while listening to its soft song. The seashell floated up to the top of the icy sea and turned northward. For many days and many nights it journeyed through the waves, all the while singing its song. And behind it swam the whales, stretched out in a long line, travelling northwards, ever northwards, past many beaches, past rocky headlands and past lighthouses.

For many days and nights they journeyed, following the song of the magic seashell. And as they journeyed, leaving the icy oceans far behind them, the water grew warmer and warmer and warmer … until one day the seashell floated into a beautiful warm bay where the blue water was so clear that the golden sunbeams could dance right through to the shining sands at the bottom.

The whales swam into the warm clear bay and knew straight away that this was the place where their babies could be born, and play together safe and warm.

The magic seashell, now that its work was done, buried itself in the shining sands at the bottom of the bay. When the Sea King looked into his treasure chest at the end of the long dark winter, there lay the magic white shell softly singing a new song …

The Bees
by Silviah Njagi

Note from Silviah: This story was written for a four-and-a-half-year-old girl whose friends were leaving our kindergarten and country (Kenya). These friends had lived on the same street with this girl and gone to the same kindergarten since she was 18 months old. She was an only child in the family and these children had become like siblings to her. The mother had related how the child had sleepless nights or would wake up crying, asking why the friends were leaving and if she would be the only one left on the street and in the kindergarten. She wanted to go to another country too. After the story the mother came back a few weeks later saying that the bee story had helped and that the child was sleeping better; though she was sad that her friends were leaving, she was now looking forward to new friends arriving. True to word, a new friend did arrive on the street and join the kindergarten, and they became good friends. I remember hearing the girl say 'Some bees went away and now we have a new bee in our hive!' This story has now become our farewell story for children leaving the kindergarten; it helps the children who are left behind as well as the ones who are leaving.

Once upon a time, in a land far, far away, there was a special beehive. The bees living there made the sweetest honey in the whole wide world.

Every morning the bees would wake up and fly together around the garden looking for the juiciest, sweetest nectar among the blossoms. The bees took their time to visit each flower in the garden, big or small.

> *Busy, busy bees are we, making lots of honey,*
> *Taking pollen from the flowers, when the day is sunny.*

The bees carried the pollen and nectar on their legs. When their sacks were heavy with pollen they would fly back to their special beehive, and scrape it all off their legs. Humming together, they would churn and mix, churn and mix, until the pollen and nectar was turned into the sweetest, most golden food in the whole wide world.

Whenever any of the bees were hurt or ill and had to stay at home, the other bees in the special beehive would take some time to take care of them.

It happened that the special beehive became very famous for its sweet, golden honey. Many bees from other parts of the world heard about it and wished they could make honey as sweet and as golden as the bees from the special beehive. What were they to do?

The fairy godmother of the bees heard the bees' special wish and decided to come to their aid. Every once in a while some bees would leave the special beehive and travel to one of the other beehives. There they would show the bees in the new hive how to churn and mix to make sweet, golden honey.

The bees left behind in the special beehive began to worry that their hive would soon be empty if many bees kept leaving. But the fairy godmother of the bees promised that whenever one or two bees left, some new bees would arrive and join the special beehive in their place. That way the special beehive was kept busy and humming with activity as the bees mixed and churned the nectar to make the sweetest, most golden honey in the whole wide world.

From this time on, the bees from the special hive lived happily together, flying out to pick the sweetest nectar and pollen until it was their turn to leave their special home and fly out to help in another hive.

Busy, busy bees are we, making lots of honey,
Taking nectar from the flowers, when the day is sunny.

The Rosella and the Strawberry Patch

The need for this story was two-fold: to encourage an anxious five-year-old child to begin to do things for himself and to discourage a parent from hovering/fussing too much. The basic idea (and the rhyme) came out of a story workshop in Sydney. The initial story idea used an owl, but as owls don't eat fruit, I have changed it from an owl to a rosella (Note: a rosella is a medium-sized Australasian parrot with a long tail and beautifully coloured plumage).

Mother Rosella lived in a large nest in the hollow of an old tree. She had a baby rosella that kept her very busy. The baby wouldn't do anything by himself, even though he had learnt how to fly and was growing into quite a big bird. Baby Rosella didn't want to leave his nest, not for anything!

When Baby Rosella was hungry he would cry out for food. Mother would say, fly with me and I will show you how to find juicy berries to eat. But the baby would sit in the nest and cry out:

I don't, I won't, I need it now!

So Mother Rosella would bring food to her baby in the nest.

When Baby Rosella was thirsty he would cry out for water. Mother would say, fly with me and I will show you how to find water to drink. But the baby would sit in the nest and cry out:

I don't, I won't, I need it now!

So Mother Rosella would bring water to her baby in the nest.

One day while Mother Rosella was sleeping in her nest through the hottest part of the afternoon, another young rosella flew by to visit. He found Baby Rosella sitting next to his mother crying out 'I am hungry. I need food now!' But Mother Rosella was fast asleep and didn't hear anything.

The new friend fluttered round the nest, calling out to Baby Rosella:

Follow me, and you will see, ripe red strawberries for our tea.

Baby Rosella called back:

I don't, I won't, I need it now!

But the new friend didn't seem to hear Baby Rosella's words, and kept fluttering round the nest and calling out:

Follow me, and you will see, ripe red strawberries for our tea.

Once again, Baby Rosella called back:

I don't, I won't, I need it now!

This time the new friend didn't wait around for any more conversation. He just continued flying through the bushland towards the strawberry patch.

Baby Rosella was left sitting in the nest, feeling quite confused. Strawberries were his favourite food, and this new friend was heading to the strawberry patch without him!

There was only one thing to do. Baby Rosella stood up, ruffled his feathers a little, and set off to fly after his new friend through the bushes – all the way to the strawberry patch.

The strawberries were ripe and sweet! And there were more berries than a rosella could count. Baby Rosella and his new friend ate their fill. Baby Rosella was enjoying himself more than he could have imagined.

When it was time to leave, the two rosellas picked some extra large berries and flew back with them through the bushland to Mother Rosella.

Then the two friends spent the rest of the afternoon playing together.

What a pleasant surprise for Mother Rosella to wake up and find some ripe red strawberries in her nest!

The Boat and the Dolphin

This story idea came out of a workshop in New Zealand. It was in response to a situation where a four-and-a-half-year-old boy found it hard to part from his parents at school drop-off time. It was suggested that the parents make a little felt dolphin (a story 'prop') to give to the child to carry all day long in his pocket while he was at school. The story could be extended with more detail about the adventures to be had on the open sea, and with a travelling song that Little Boat sings as it follows the dolphin out to sea and back again.

There was once a Little Boat that lived in the safe, calm harbour.

Little Boat had a special friend – a silver dolphin who came to visit her every day. The silver dolphin would dive around Little Boat and tell of adventures on the open sea – the whales that were as big as ships, the coloured fish and all the different sea birds.

Little Boat had watched other boats go out to sea each day, and wanted to go with them and have adventures, but was not sure about leaving the safe harbour.

One day Little Boat told her thoughts to her friend the silver dolphin. The dolphin promised to guide Little Boat out to the open sea and then guide Little Boat all the way home. Little Boat followed the silver dolphin out to sea and had a wonderful journey. Little Boat saw many new things – the whales that were as big as ships, the coloured fish and all the different sea birds.

Little Boat discovered that she especially loved riding with the winds, this way and that – and sometimes the winds would even help blow Little Boat all the way home, and the silver dolphin had to swim very fast to keep up!

From this time on Little Boat travelled out to the open sea every day. And every night the winds, together with the silver dolphin, would guide Little Boat home again.

The Not-So-Perfect House

This story was written for a ten-year-old boy who was very anxious about things needing to always be perfect – the ending was left for him to accept as finished or to complete with his own ideas. This story could be adapted for girls by changing the main character to a woman. However it is not a story just for children – an adult friend of mine who heard this story commented that it spoke directly to him!

There was once a perfect man who lived in a perfect house and had a perfect life – or so he thought! Every day he would do his perfect work, sweeping his floor, dusting his shelves, washing his clothes, polishing his boots.

As he worked he would sing his perfect song:

A perfect life is the life for me, a perfect house is the place to be!

There was not a spot of dust anywhere in the life of this perfect man. There was not one thing out of place in the life of this perfect man. The only slight hiccup was that, because the perfect man was always worrying about things needing to be perfect, he didn't sleep very well at night.

One day, when the perfect man had lifted up a rug to clean underneath it, he discovered a small door in the floor. He pulled open the new door and saw stairs going down into a room deep in the ground under his perfect house. He had never known about this room before! With torch in hand, he carefully climbed down the stairs to explore this new discovery. To his surprise, the under-floor room was empty, except for one thing. In the middle of the floor was a large wooden chest with a wooden lid and a large metal lock. But there was no key in sight.

The perfect man tried many ways to get the chest open but the lock was too strong. So he had to leave the wooden chest down in the new room and return upstairs to get on with his perfect life. There was sweeping and dusting to be done!

Some days passed, but the perfect man couldn't stop wondering what was in the large wooden chest. In fact he could hardly sleep at night because of wondering. Finally he took a torch and a hammer and went down the stairs into the under-floor room. He was going to get that chest open no matter what! He banged the lock with his hammer until the lock broke and the lid sprang open.

In the light of his torch the man could see a very old pillow, a very big pillow, a pillow just about as big as he was! This pillow had been tightly squashed into the box for a very long time but now was free to burst out.

The pillow burst out with a rip and a puff – and out of the pillow came flying a million tiny feathers. They went up the man's nose (ah-choo!) and covered him from top to toe. They travelled up the stairs and into the house and filled every room. They travelled out the windows and doors and filled up his garden.

There were feathers, feathers, everywhere! The man chased them with his broom and his dusting cloth (ah-choo!), but the feathers just flew up in the air and settled down elsewhere. The man went outside and chased them with his garden rake but the feathers flew up in the air and settled down elsewhere.

After many hours of chasing feathers the man was exhausted. He lay down to sleep on his feather-covered bed. To his surprise, he had the most comfortable sleep of his whole life.

(NOTE – this story could be completed in a few different ways by the writer or the listener 'The next morning when the man woke up, he had an idea … ' Or the story could be left as it is.)

'Story bones' – The Not-So-Perfect Car/ The Not-So-Perfect Garden

In workshops in Tasmania, on the south coast of NSW and another in China, several groups discussed the challenge of children, usually primary school age and older (even adults) who get extremely anxious because they always want things to be perfect. Many different groups worked a storyline on this theme, with the message that things don't have to be 'perfect' to get the job done. I have included the 'story bones' of two of these groups below for you to flesh out into full stories.

The Not-So-Perfect Car

A mechanic makes a convertible car out of many bits and pieces – he 'tinkered and tuckered, blinkered and blockered' but things didn't fit quite right – the car worked but not perfectly. This story had many possible endings, with the car helping to rescue someone or something, or the car being used to transport people out of town before the river rose in the flood, etc. – in other words, the car served a good purpose even if it was not 'perfect'.

The Not-So-Perfect Garden

A gardener who expected everything in her garden to be 'just so' – all her flowers in perfect rows, her vegetables growing to perfect heights, her garden walls always very straight and smooth – she would walk around each day inspecting everything – if things weren't going well, 'her face fell and she let out a yell!'

One day a storm passed over with a wind so strong that it knocked down one of her garden walls. She tried to rebuild it but the rocks did not fit together perfectly – she became very angry and stormed off for a walk – soon she arrived at a river and sat on the bank throwing sticks into the water – then she noticed a beaver diving and picking up every stick that she threw into the river – the beaver swam with the stick and put it into his dam wall – no matter what kind of stick the gardener threw in, straight or curly, long or short, heavy or light, the beaver found a use for it.

'I can do this' thought the gardener – and she stood up and walked back home and continued with building her wall, using every kind of stone she could find – round or long, heavy or light, large or small – and by the end of her work she had built the strongest rock wall in the town.

5

Bullying/Exclusion/Teasing

Clever Chameleon

A Meru Story from Kenya, by Silviah Njagi. A wonderful story for five- to ten-year-olds with the theme of overcoming teasing and bullying behaviour

> *Nderirwe ni baba, Ndijage Kaora, Ntikeje Kuomora, Ndiguru*
> (My father told me to walk slowly so that I do not cause the earth to break)

In a great jungle there lived a chameleon and all the other animals like elephant, cheetah, monkey and lion. Chameleon liked to lie on a branch and roll his big eyes from side to side as he waited for flies to fly nearby and then he would roll out his tongue and catch them. Sometimes he would walk slowly on the grass while he sang 'nde, nde, nderirwe ... '

All the large animals teased chameleon for they thought he walked too slowly. They even said he was weak and his legs would probably break one day. Chameleon, however, just ate his flies and rolled his eyes from side to side and kept singing his song 'nde, nde, nderirwe ... '

One day, while chameleon was lying on a branch and rolling his eyes from side to side, elephant appeared. Without even a word of hello he said to chameleon in a big trumpety sound: 'I have heard that you sing about how you walk slowly because you do not want to break the earth! I want you to know that I, elephant, am the strongest animal in the jungle, and I can break the earth ten times more than anyone else. At sunrise tomorrow, I will summon all the animals to gather around the great Muringa tree and I will show everyone that you are not as strong as I am.

I AM THE ELEPHANT!'

After saying this, elephant walked away, laughing with his great big trumpety voice that echoed through the whole jungle.

Chameleon sat on his branch, rolling his eyes from side to side. He tried to sing but only a whisper came: 'Nde, nde, nderirwe … '

Then chameleon remembered his friend the mole-rat. Mole-rat liked to make burrows and pathways under the earth. The only way to tell where mole-rat was at work was to look for big heaps of earth that he left as he dug. Chameleon spotted mole-rat's last heap of earth and hurried as fast as he could to reach it. When he arrived he called to his friend, 'Mole-rat, mole-rat, it's me, chameleon. Come out for I would like to speak to you.'

As soon as mole-rat came out of his burrow, chameleon said, 'Elephant has challenged me to break the earth at sunrise tomorrow, and I need your help.'

Together chameleon and mole rat walked slowly to the great Muringa tree. They sang chameleon's song in whispers, as they did not want to be heard: 'Nde, nde, nderirwe … '

Mole-rat burrowed under the earth while chameleon carried away the heap of earth to hide under a bush. By the time they had finished, the first cock was crowing and it was nearly sunrise. Mole-rat wished good luck to his friend chameleon and dug his way back to his usual burrow.

Chameleon waited as he sang 'Nde, nde, nderirwe … '

As the sun spread its first rays over the jungle, the animals began to gather around the great Muringa tree. Then at last the elephant came. Because chameleon was already there and had chosen his side of the tree, elephant took the other side and had to be first to try to break the earth. Elephant lifted his big paw and bought it crashing down to the earth with a loud thud, but nothing happened. He tried again and again, but still the earth did not crack. When he was tired and sweating and could lift his paw no more, it was chameleon's turn.

Chameleon knew exactly where mole-rat had dug the burrow under the earth so he lifted his thin leg as high as he could and brought it down with a quiet step. And as soon as his leg touched the earth, it began to crack, and crack, and crack … until there was a big hole in the ground.

All the animals cheered chameleon and from that day onwards no one teased him or laughed at him. They all joined him in his song and dance: 'Nde, nde, nderirwe … '

Rainbow Colours
by Janine Hutton

Following a therapeutic storytelling workshop in Moruya, this story was written by a parent for the four- and five-year-old children attending the local playgroup. Her aim was twofold: to address an out-of-balance 'exclusivity' that had arisen with some 'pushing behaviour', and also to address this behaviour itself.

Note from the author: I have finally put the story onto paper. However it has been a little different each time I have told it. When I told it to the group I seemed to read the mood of the day and the moment, and repeat certain parts of the story or embellish when appropriate.

The story has been lovely. The children seem to have really enjoyed it. One child looked for rainbow clothes to wear to playgroup, while another said 'We have to go to playgroup today as Janine is telling the rainbow story.' Others repeated parts of it during free play.

We certainly seem to have made some changes to play and 'exclusiveness' at playgroup. I think this was really a mix of a number of strategies. The story seemed to have a special quality – maybe just the simple essence of working together (three parents worked on the initial idea) and writing it especially for our children.

It was a still spring morning when all of a sudden the wind started to blow. It grew stronger and stronger, blowing dark clouds across the sky.

All the birds and other little animals were out foraging for food when they noticed it was getting darker and darker.

There was lightning and thunder and the rain came tumbling down. It was so dark all the colours of the world became very dull and almost impossible to see.

The birds were chirping very loudly to each other and all the animals were trying to find their way home.

The darker it got the duller the colours became and the harder it was for the animals to find their way home.

Mother Nature was very worried: she knew it was important for all the colours to be bright enough to see, so she thought and she thought and she thought.

Then it came to her. Once the storm had settled and the sun came back out, a rainbow in the sky would show all the colours how to be bright and play and work together again.

Mother Nature was right! Once the sun came back out there was a beautiful rainbow in the sky and all the colours shone brightly and all the birds and animals found their way home.

The story was followed each time by a wooden rainbow puzzle game – some children were individually invited to come and place a piece of coloured block in the rainbow puzzle to build a rainbow together as the group sang a rainbow song.

The Golden Dolphin

This story was written for a six-year-old boy who always wanted to be the centre of attention, and was continually trying to exclude others from his play. It was presented as a puppet show at pre-school (and the child loved to act this out in free play). A copy was given to his parents to read to him at bedtime. The story was intended for both parents and child.

There was once a dolphin who loved the sun. She spent all her time leaping up above the waves to play in the sunlight. One time she leapt so high that she was able to catch a golden sunbeam and wrap it round herself like a shiny golden coat. From this time on she was known by all her dolphin friends as the golden dolphin, and her friends lived in wonder of her golden light.

You may think that this golden dolphin was a healthy, happy dolphin. But in spending all her time leaping up high above the waves, she was missing out on diving down deep with her dolphin friends and exploring the blue waters below – something that all dolphins need to do.

Her friends tried to encourage her to dive with them but the golden dolphin was not interested. She would just keep leaping up into the sunshine and skimming across the waves and leaping up again. She had even learnt to catch the fish that came close to the surface of the water, so she never needed to dive down deep for her food.

One day the golden dolphin was leaping and dancing across the waves when she saw ahead of her a beautiful rainbow. The golden dolphin had seen rainbows before, and had even tried to leap up and catch the rainbow colours – but they always disappeared when she swam too close.

But this rainbow was different. This rainbow stretched down below the surface of the water – down, down, down, into the dark ocean below. When the golden dolphin leapt across the waves to get closer, she could see the colour paths reaching deep into the water. The colours were so beautiful and they were calling out, 'Follow me'!

Follow me and you will see, colours deep beneath the sea, colours blue and colours green, red, purple and orange – like you've never seen!

At first the golden dolphin was frightened to dive down deep, but she found that if she stayed close to the colour paths then she always felt safe. The first colour path she followed was a red one and this led her to a wonderful garden of red coral. The second colour path was an orange one and this led her to some orange starfish lying in the sand deep down at the bottom of the sea. The next colour path was a green one and this led her into a thick bed of seaweed where the green weed swayed gently to and fro. The other colour paths took her to parts of the ocean where many purple and blue and yellow fish were playing, and she had such fun chasing them in and out of the coral gardens and the swaying seaweed.

What a wonderful underwater world the golden dolphin had discovered!

It wasn't long before the other dolphins joined the golden dolphin, diving down together to explore the deep blue sea. The golden dolphin soon discovered that her golden coat would light up the waters wherever she was swimming so there was no place too dark or too deep for her to explore. And every once in a while the golden dolphin would leap up high above the waves to catch some golden sunlight before diving down deep once again, as all dolphins like to do!

> Dive dolphin dive, dive down into the deep blue water, leap up to catch the golden sunlight,
> dive down into the deep blue water, dive dolphin dive!

Baba Simba

This story idea was shared in a workshop in Kenya by an African male teacher with a deep booming voice. It completely captivated the fifty people in the room (the power of the storyteller!) It drew its theme from a traditional Kenyan folktale. The teacher wanted a strong story for a nine-year-old boy in his class who was continually being mean and bullying the others. 'Baba Simba' is Kiswahili for 'Father Lion'.

Baba Simba lived in the forest, in a lush grassy home by the river. The forest was Baba Simba's kingdom and all the animals worked for him. He was the King of the Forest!

In his kingdom, Baba Simba insisted that every animal that lived in the forest had to bring him a share of their food. This way Baba Simba didn't have to do any work.

Each day the animals would line up outside Baba Simba's home to give their share. Baba Simba would grab the food greedily and never give thanks to anyone.

One day Fox decided he had had enough of Baba Simba's mean and greedy ways. He had had enough of giving his food to a mean and greedy lion, and so he decided to play a trick on him.

Fox told Baba Simba that he was on the path by the river when another Baba Simba jumped out of the water and took his contribution. There was nothing Fox could do so he had come without any food to give to Baba Simba.

Baba Simba was very angry that another lion had come to live in his forest. He went straight to the river's edge to look for this other Baba Simba, and when he looked into the water he saw a great big lion staring up at him.

Straight away, Baba Simba jumped into the water to fight this other lion. He bashed around in the river, hitting out at rocks and floating tree branches and anything else he could find to hit, but he couldn't find the other lion anywhere.

Then Baba Simba looked back up to the riverbank and saw Fox and all the other forest animals. They were pointing at him and laughing at him. He realized that he had been tricked, and he climbed out of the water feeling very embarrassed and ashamed. In his shame he sent all the animals away, and from that time on Baba Simba used his own strength to do his own hunting.

Bully Bear
by Aimee Chua

Aimee flew from the Philippines to attend my workshop in Singapore. She then returned to her therapy work back in Oloilo City and wrote this story for a seven-year-old boy who was bullying his classmates and being cruel to animals. He had started to blame other children when he was caught misbehaving, and he was having difficulty staying friends with his classmates and cousins. The boy was the middle child in a family of three sons. The story was told to him by his mother and he kept asking her to repeat it! The mother reported that the story had been very soothing and helpful for him.

Once upon a time there lived a family of bears in the forest. There was mama bear, papa bear and three little baby bears. This particular family of bears was special. When each of the three little baby bears was born, the wind blew through the trees and whispered that each baby bear was given a special gift for him to discover and use wisely.

The years passed in peace and plenty and the three little bears grew tall and strong. Unbeknown to them, the animals and trees of the forest kept watch as the bears frolicked and rambled all through the wide woodland. The creatures of the forest made sure that the little bears didn't fall into the ravine nor drown in the deep blue river nor lose their way in the swamplands where crocodiles hunted.

As each little bear grew big and strong he learnt to master and perfect his gift. All except one little bear!

He was the little bear who could lift boulders, throw huge logs across the air, and crumple the hardest iron in his bare fist. He could haul firewood for mama bear's fire but he could also step on squirrel's feet in anger. He could carry a sick little elephant home to its family but he could also make hippo's head twinge when he struck him during play. He could do just about any task that needed brute force; but was extraordinary strength his great gift?

Little Bear asked himself this question every time he made his friends cry or caused his mother's face to grow sad. 'Is extraordinary strength indeed the great gift given me?' he'd ask.

Little Bear was sitting alone on a rock beside the deep blue river asking this same question when a little turtle nibbled on his toe. Little Bear was about to throw a rock at the turtle when a sudden gust of wind toppled him into the deep blue river. Oh! How Little Bear spluttered and struggled and tried to keep his head above the water. Bears know how to swim but the weeds growing thickly in the riverbanks had caught around Little Bear's legs.

Little Bear thought all was lost until he noticed Turtle gnawing at the hardy reeds binding his legs. He stopped thrashing and finally heard Turtle say, 'The water isn't deep little bear, only your fears are deceiving you. Keep still and you will soon be free'. Turtle kept on gnawing at the stubborn reeds until Little Bear could climb once more onto the rock beside the river.

Little Bear remembered how he tried to throw a rock at Turtle for nibbling on his toe. Shyly he asked turtle, 'Why did you help me when I tried to throw a rock at you?'

Turtle laughed and told Little Bear, 'I also remembered the times when you played with me even when I was slow. You carried me on your back when I couldn't climb a tree. You shared your bananas with me when I knew those bananas were not enough to feed a hungry little bear. You have a great capacity to care and for this I saved you.'

Turtle's words brought understanding to Little Bear. He finally learned that caring for others was his great gift.

Hot Hippo

A Kikuyu tale from East Africa, transcribed by Susan Perrow. A wonderful story for all ages about how Ngai, the great God of Everything, finds a way for a large animal like a hippopotamus to safely share the river with even the smallest of fish.

Hippo was hot and Hippo was dusty.

He sat on the riverbank and gazed at all the fish swimming in the water. They must be so so cool, he thought to himself. If only I could live in the water, how cool and wonderful life would be.

Hippo decided to visit Ngai who was the god of everything and everywhere, and see if he could help with an answer to his problem. It was Ngai who had told the animals to live on the land and the fishes to live in the water. It was Ngai who had told the birds to fly in the air and the ants to live under the ground. It was Ngai who had told Hippo he was to live on the land and eat grass.

So Hippo walked and walked across the grassy plains, getting hotter with every step he took, and mumbling to himself as he went along:

> *I'm hot, hot, hot, and I'm not, not, not, getting cool any way:*
> *I'm dusty and I'm hot, and I know just what, would make me cooler each day.*

He walked and he walked over many hills, getting hotter with every step he took, and mumbling to himself as he went along:

> *I'm hot, hot, hot, and I'm not, not, not, getting cool any way:*
> *I'm dusty and I'm hot, and I know just what, would make me cooler each day.*

He walked and he walked through the forests of acacia trees, getting hotter with every step he took, and mumbling to himself as he went along:

> *I'm hot, hot, hot, and I'm not, not, not, getting cool any way:*
> *I'm dusty and I'm hot, and I know just what, would make me cooler each day.*

He walked and he walked and he walked, until he came to the mountain where Ngai lived.

'Please, O great Ngai, God of Everything and everywhere, I would so much like to live in the water and not on the dry land,' called out Hippo hopefully. 'But I promise that I would still eat grass.'

'Aha!' sung out the voice of Ngai from the mountain top. 'So you say. But one day you might, just might, eat a fish to see if it tasted good. And then you might eat ALL MY LITTLE FISHES!'

'Oh no, I promise I wouldn't,' said Hippo. 'Aha!' sung out the voice of Ngai. 'So you say! But how can I be sure of that? I love my little fishes!'

'I would show you,' promised Hippo. 'I will let you look in my mouth whenever you like, to see that I am not eating your little fishes. And I will stir up the water with my tail so you can see I have not hidden the bones.'

'Aha!' sung out the voice of Ngai. 'Then you may live in the water but … ' Hippo waited … 'But you must come out on to the land at night and eat grass, so that even in the dark I can tell you are not eating my little fishes. Agreed?'

Hippo happily agreed and he quickly walked all the way home (as fast as his little legs could carry him) through the acacia forests, over many hills, and across the grassy plains. When he got to the river he jumped in with a mighty SPLASH! He sank like a stone and because he couldn't swim he held his breath and ran along the bottom.

And to this day you will find Hippo on the bottom of the water by day and eating grass on the land by night. In the day he stirs up the bottom by wagging his little tail, so that Ngai can see he has not hidden any fish-bones. And now and then he floats to the top of the pool and opens his huge mouth ever so wide and says: 'Look, Ngai! No fishes!'

And if you listen carefully, you may hear him in the river pools singing his 'cooling' song:

I'm cool, cool, cool, living in this pool, I'm so very cool everyday!

King Flower

This story idea was thought up by a group of Chinese teachers in Shenzhen. It was devised as a creative strategy for a seven-year-old girl who was 'slow' in her development, and quite sensitive about this. All the other children were making fun of her. This is an example of a story written for victims of bullying and teasing. One would hope that teasers and bullies would also be touched by such a story.

There was once a Chinese princess who lived with her parents in a beautiful palace. This princess had everything she could wish for, except friends. Days and weeks and months would go by without the young girl having anyone to play with.

Her father the king noticed that his daughter was lonely and so he organized a grand party for her. The king invited many young girls from across the land to the party and asked each one of them to bring the most beautiful plant they could find to present as a gift to his daughter.

Eventually the day of the party arrived. The invited guests came into the palace carrying all kinds of pots with beautiful flowering plants. But one of the girls was carrying a pot with only a small shoot coming out from the soil. When the other children saw this they all laughed. 'What a silly little plant,' they cried out. 'Imagine bringing this as a gift – it doesn't even have a flower!'

The king asked for all the pots to be put in a large circle for the princess to choose her favourite one. The princess walked slowly past all the pots, looking carefully at each of the flowering plants. Eventually she pointed to the pot with the tiny shoot. 'This is my favourite one,' she said, 'as it still has room and time to grow.'

From that day on, the girl who had brought the pot with the tiny shoot was invited back to the palace to play every day with the princess. Together they cared for the tiny shoot and after many days the shoot grew into a tall and healthy plant with 'king flowers' – the largest and most beautiful of all the flowers in China.

'Story bones' – The Dolphin and the Storm

This story idea came from a group of teachers in Noosa Heads, Queensland. It was for a seven-year-old boy who was not included by the group.

A pod of dolphins swimming near coral reef – a storm hits – one dolphin is tossed against reef, cut and bruised, then caught in a riptide – eventually dolphin gives up fighting against the current and flows with it – he meets an old dolphin who shows him the way back to the group – and on the way the older, wiser dolphin teaches the younger one some new ways of catching fish. When the younger dolphin rejoins the pod he shows the others his new tricks.

6

Death/Dying/Illness

Heavenly Magic

A story for Tao Tao

A story written for a five-year-old boy whose father had died by drowning the previous year. I met with the mother to find out more about the boy: his favourite things — toys, animals, things he liked to do. One of his favourite story books was about a bunny rabbit, and his favourite item, since he was a toddler, was his bunny blanket. I had also observed the boy in kindergarten and could see that he had a very close connection to his 'bunny blanket'. He took it with him everywhere, and whenever the slightest thing upset him he would wrap himself in it. His mother was planning to move to a new country where her son would be enrolled in a new school. She believed it was important for him to be able to start 'big' (primary/elementary) school without his blanket (to avoid him being teased), but to date all her attempts to lessen the dependence on the blanket had been unsuccessful. The intention of this story was twofold — to aid metamorphosis of his security blanket into two special carry bags (one for him and one for his toy rabbits), and to help build a link between the boy and the place where the boy and his mother believed his father had passed on to (heaven). In a window of time when the boy had gone on an outing without the blanket, the mother planned for it to be sewn into the two bags, and some spare scraps of it used to make a blanket jacket for his toy rabbit. When the boy returned home, there would be a gift wrapped in special 'starry' paper waiting on his bed, with the story rolled up in a scroll (tied with golden thread).

There was once a special blanket that belonged to a little boy called Tao Tao. This boy loved his blanket so much that he slept with it every night, and took it with him everywhere he went. The blanket was his friend, and Tao Tao was the blanket's friend. They were happy together.

For many years the blanket liked this special friendship, but as Tao Tao grew older, it became quite difficult for the blanket to follow him everywhere. Tao Tao, like all growing boys, loved to climb trees and jump puddles and ride high on the swing, and the blanket was getting too old and too tired to do all these things. But the blanket still wanted to be Tao Tao's friend, and wanted to be a help to him as he was growing up into a tall strong boy.

Tao Tao's father looked down from high in heaven, and also wanted to find a way to help. At last he had an idea. He worked some heavenly magic to turn the blanket into a blanket bag, a bag that could easily travel with Tao Tao wherever he went. This new bag could carry Tao Tao's special things – his toys and his crayons and his books.

And, as an extra surprise, when Tao Tao's father worked his special magic, there was enough cloth left to make some tiny jackets for Tao Tao's new toy rabbits – a baby jacket for baby rabbit and a daddy jacket for daddy rabbit. The rabbits loved to live inside the blanket bag, and they all became friends together.

The Oriole and the Cherry Tree

Singapore: a story for a primary school where one of the pupils had died in a car accident. The plan for the story was to tell it at assembly to all the children as part of the memorial service – the school had a cherry tree in the garden, hence the choice of this tree in the story. The girl who had died was very popular with all the students, and a leader figure in the school.

There was once a beautiful cherry tree that grew in the middle of a large garden where many birds and insects flew and fluttered and flitted. Children loved to play in the shade of the cherry tree. They especially loved it in the summer when the branches were laden with ripe, red, juicy cherries.

The cherry tree enjoyed all the birds and insects and children who played around it, but it had one special friend, a golden oriole bird. This beautiful bird had its nest on one of the tree's top branches and from here it sang sweetly all day.

But it happened one night, without any warning, that a violent storm passed over the garden. There was lightning and thunder and strong winds and rain. One of the lightning flashes hit the top branch of the cherry tree and killed the golden oriole bird in an instant.

The storm passed over, leaving the cherry tree and all the garden friends mourning the death of the golden bird. The cherry tree was so upset at the loss of its friend that it refused to flower the next spring – and without any flowers there would be no cherries in the summer.

The bees that liked to get pollen from the cherry tree flowers circled the tree and hummed a special song to the tree. Soon all the other friends from the garden joined in the song … the ants, dragonflies, butterflies, birds and children …

The song helped the cherry tree find the strength to grow its flowers once again, and the following summer it was covered with ripe, red, juicy cherries.

(Note: the children were encouraged to go back to class to help their teacher write the words for a related song; then at the next assembly each class sang its song for the rest of the school.)

Grandfather's Cloak of Light

A story for use with young children when their grandparents or elderly relatives have died.

Grandfather was sitting in his favourite chair in the garden, thinking back to all the beautiful moments in his life. It was almost time for him to set off on the long path back to heaven. Around him the butterflies and birds flitted in and out the rays of golden sunlight, weaving a special cloak of light for grandfather to wear on his journey.

By the end of the day the sun was ready to go to bed and let the moon take her turn in the sky. Grandfather was still outside. The garden chair was so comfortable that he had fallen asleep.

Mother Moon shone down her silver light and the night spirits wove some of her light into Grandfather's cloak. Then all the little stars took a turn, and shone down an extra sparkle and twinkle into the cloak.

When the cloak of light was ready, Grandfather woke up, wrapped it tightly around his tired old shoulders, and set off on his journey.

As he was crossing the sky, he remembered to stop, just for a moment, to blow a kiss back down to all his family. The dawn clouds caught the kiss in their early morning colours and when grandfather's family woke up they could see it shimmering in the sunrise.

The Butterfly

Rewritten from an anonymous source by Susan Perrow – a story about death, life and transformation, for children aged four and upwards. This is especially beautiful when presented as a puppet show – I usually tell it with a green cloth over my lap (for the garden) and some puppets made from coloured combed fleece: the caterpillar starts off very small, with new and larger ones hiding in the folds of the cloth as he eats and grows bigger.

With tired wings an old butterfly once fluttered over a field. It made its way towards a green bush and laid a tiny egg under a leaf and crawled away.

The egg was left in the care of Mother Earth. During the day the sun warmed it from above; at night the earth warmed it from below. The leaf protected it from rain, and so it was well cared for. The glow of life of the old butterfly had gone out, but in its egg lived a spark.

Already after only a few days there was a gentle movement under the delicate skin. A sunbeam played around the green leaf of the plant, calling, 'Come out, come out.' There was a pulling and stretching in the egg, the skin tore, and out came a tiny yellow caterpillar, covered with little dots and with skin as smooth as silk.

The little creature crawled towards a green leaf, which then became its garden, house and food. The edge of the leaf was especially good to eat and the tiny caterpillar began to gnaw out little corners. After a few days almost all this leaf was gone, and the sunbeam said, 'It's time to find your way into the wide green world.'

So the caterpillar began its journey, crawling from bush to bush, from leaf to leaf. As it crawled it munched, and as it munched it grew. It crawled and munched, it munched and grew. Soon the tiny caterpillar had grown into a very large caterpillar.

By this time summer was coming to an end and the autumn winds were blowing across the fields and through the bushes. The sunlight seemed to say, 'Find a quiet place to rest.'

The caterpillar crawled down between some rocks into a dark and quiet space. Mother Earth wrapped it in her warm arms, and the caterpillar fell into a deep sleep. While it slept, through the long winter, delicate elves wove a special gown for it. With their mysterious fingers they wove the sparkle of the stars and the glow of the rainbow into the cloak.

Spring came, and brought some sunny days. The warmth of the sun reached deep into the earth. While flowers were opening to the light above ground, a butterfly was waking up below the ground. The caterpillar had died, but in its place a butterfly was climbing up through a crack in the rocks, climbing up towards the light. It could hear the flower song and it could feel the warmth of the spring sunbeams.

It opened its beautiful new wings and flew up high.

A Doll from Heaven

A story for Esther's kindergarten children

Note: Teacher Esther died unexpectedly on the way home from school one day. She was only 33 and had been teaching in the Mbagathi Kindergarten, Nairobi, for 9 years. This story was told in English and Kiswahili to the children every day for a week after Esther's death. A display was set up in a corner of the room using a backdrop of blue, and a simple marionette doll was hung in the blue 'sky'. This was made from brown silk and a white headcloth embroidered with gold and silver threads. The children absorbed the story so deeply that they told their parents they didn't need to be sad any more – Teacher Esther was watching over them every day!

After a long journey across the blue sky, Teacher Esther was safe in heaven. She was happy to be back with God's angels – her work in the world was completed for now.

At night, in the light of the twinkling stars, she could see down to earth and see her kindergarten children asleep in their beds in their homes. In the daytime, when the sun was shining brightly, she could see down to the kindergarten where her children were playing together. She was so happy that they had a new teacher to take care of them.

But Teacher Esther could also see that her children were missing her and were feeling sad. So she decided to send down a gift from heaven – a little doll to watch over her children in their kindergarten room.

And so, with her large basket, Teacher Esther set out to cross the heavens, gathering golden threads from the sun and silver threads from the moon. When her basket was full with threads, she wove a special cloth on her heavenly loom to make a doll.

When the doll was ready, one of heaven's angels cradled it in her wings and set out to travel across the sky of twinkling stars and down to earth. When the angel arrived at the kindergarten she reached in through the window and hung the doll just above the story table so all the children would find it in the morning.

The next day when the children arrived at the kindergarten they found their new friend waiting to greet them. The doll sparkled gold and silver in the morning light and the children were so happy to see her. The children knew it was a heavenly gift and from that day onwards the little doll watched over their play and smiled down on them each day.

The Tortoise and the Market Bus

In a workshop with 'Médecins Sans Frontières' in Kenya, a group of nurses wrote the following story for patients who are late for appointments or in denial of their illness, or who bring their children late for appointments or are in denial of their children's illness. The story was deliberately kept short so the nurses could share it with each patient. The patients were encouraged to change 'market' to 'clinic' in the little rhyme.

There was once a village where many animals lived and worked. This village was far away from any markets. Once a week a bus came to pick up all the animals so they could go to market to buy food.

Mr Tortoise however was quite a lazy fellow and would often miss the bus. Then he would beg all the other animals for food to eat. Soon he was known as the 'village beggar'.

The animals had a meeting about this and decided that each one should take a turn to wake Mr Tortoise on the day of the bus so he would be able to catch it and do his own shopping. The animals at the meeting made up a song:

> *Wake up! wake up! It's market day. Wake up! The bus is on its way,*
> *Wake up or you'll be late today, wake up to join our trip today.*

So from this time on, with the help of the other village animals, Mr Tortoise always woke in time to catch the market bus and didn't have to beg again.

The Hare, the Parrot and the Bear

A story to help patients understand and cope with 'opportunistic infections'.

In a workshop with 'Médecins Sans Frontières' in Nairobi, a group of counsellors wrote the following story to help Aids patients (children and adults) understand and cope with 'opportunistic infections'. The group identified the following metaphors: the hare's children are the clients, the

*bear is the 'opportunistic infection', the parrot is the witch doctor or priest
(who are often anti-Aids and anti-help), and the mother's song and the
helping 'peephole' represent the doctors and counsellors.*

A mother hare lived in a house in the forest with her children. Every
day the mother hare needed to go out to hunt for food. To make sure
her little ones were safe, she taught them a song to listen for so they
would know it was their mother at the door and not a stranger.

One day a hungry bear came to the door and knocked. The children called out, 'If you are our mother, please sing us your song.' The
bear was angry at this and stomped back into the forest. A parrot that
lived in the tree was watching and flew after the bear and offered to
teach him the mother's song.

The bear returned and sang the song. At first the children were confused
as this voice was quite low and husky, so they still refused to open the door.
The bear kept singing many times until the children decided it must be
their mother and opened the door to them. The bear caught and ate one
of the little hares and wandered off back into the forest.

When the mother hare returned she was very upset and decided
to trick the bear so he could never catch any more of her children.
She found a strong stick and poked a small peephole in the door, just
big enough for the little children to see through. From this time on
whenever the bear returned the children could see exactly who it was
and never ever opened their door again to anyone except their mother.

The Rainbow Dove

*A story for a special friend who recently lost her 25-year-old daughter in
a fire. This story was shared amongst the extended family, especially to
give some positive images to the young children.*

There was once a beautiful white dove who always wanted to fly up
high. Instead of spending her time foraging for food and playing in
and out of the branches of the forest with all the other doves, she was
more interested in exploring the secrets of the sky.

Eventually the white dove flew so high that she reached the top of the
rainbow. There she met the rainbow spirit who taught her the wisdom of
the colours. Using this new wisdom, the white dove was able to change
all her white wing feathers to rainbow ones. She was so happy!

The white dove flew back down to the forest and in and out of the trees, leaving some of her new, bright feathers for family and friends to find … colourful treasure-feathers that would last for ever.

Then the white dove flapped her rainbow wings and flew up high in the sky to meet the sun.

The King and his Three Sons

This is an anonymous story, rewritten by Susan Perrow, which has been passed down from storyteller to storyteller. It has a positive message of light, hope and simplicity, and the universal theme of a father or mother passing on, and another filling his/her space. It can figure either sons or daughters. Suitable for ages 5–10.

There was once a king who was very ill. He knew he didn't have many more days to live and he was trying to decide which of his three sons was the wisest, and could be left in charge of ruling his kingdom. So he devised a task; and whichever son best fulfilled the task would be his chosen heir.

He took each son to a room – each was empty and exactly the same size – and he gave them a riddle for their task.

> *Fill this room from roof to floor*
> *Fill it till it can be filled no more*
> *Leave no spaces to be seen*
> *Leave no spaces in between*
> *Do this task within one day*
> *And then upon my throne you'll stay.*

Then the king left each son with his empty room, telling them he would be back in one day.

The first brother thought, 'I'll fill my room with rocks, great big rocks.' He ordered his servants to start bringing in wagonloads of rocks from the king's quarry. Soon huge rocks were piled on the floor to fill the room … but what about the spaces in between?

The second brother thought, 'There is plenty of wheat ready in the fields to be harvested – I'll fill my room with stalks of wheat.' So he ordered the farmers to bring in cartloads of wheat. The room seemed to fill up quickly … but what about the spaces in between?

The third brother thought for a while, then he knew exactly what to do. He spent the morning doing other tasks, ate some soup and bread for lunch, and then took two things into the room – in less than a second the room was full … completely full!

And the third brother was made heir to the kingdom and he ruled it wisely and justly for the rest of his life.

What were the two things the third brother took into the room? *(See answer upside down below)*

Answer: ꓕ ɔɐuɐlɔ ɐuq ɐ pox oɟ ɯɐʇɔɥǝs

'Story bones' – The Marathon Runner

In a workshop with 'Médecins Sans Frontières' in Nairobi, a group of counsellors came up with the following story idea for Aids patients (children and adults) who suffer from 'treatment fatigue'. Apparently it is quite a common occurrence for patients to forget (or not to bother, or not think it is important) to take their pills every day. The story was deliberately kept short so the nurses giving out the medicine could share it with each patient, but it could be worked on to build up the tension with more detail and a longer journey.

A marathon runner is given a task to circle the world. He knows it will be a very long journey so he packs many things into his survival bag to help him on his way (strong shoes, a fire stick, a long rope).

His first obstacle is a river to cross. As he is trying to decide how to do this a lion comes out of the bushes and roars at him. Somehow the fear of the lion gives him the strength to jump right over the river, from one bank to the other.

He continues on his way. Soon he reaches a mountain range but he can hear elephants coming towards him. He lights his fire stick and flashes it at them and they run off. After successfully scaring away the elephants he is filled with the strength to climb over the mountains. He puts on his strong climbing shoes and sets off up the rocky cliffs.

On the other side he finds the ocean and here he meets a fast swimming dolphin. He uses his rope to catch the dolphin and then climbs on his new friend's back; and together they travel the rest of the journey, across the sea and back home again, having many more adventures on his ocean crossing!

7

Disrespect/Lack of Care
(self/others/things)

A Day in the Life of my Hat

The idea for this poem, and the first few lines, came from a workshop in St Kilda, Melbourne as a playful response to four-year-old children not wanting to wear hats outside. In the hot Australian summer climate, wearing hats is important for self-care and this habit needs to be learned at an early age. The group thought it would be fun to have a funny approach to encouraging hat wearing, as an alternative to continual 'boring' reminders.

My hat for my head
Waits on the hat peg
When I play outside
My hat comes for a ride.

My head is the horse,
Pretending of course!
My hat rides it around
As I run on the ground.

When I go down the slide
My hat loves this fun ride!
Together we play
Till the end of the day

Then my hat comes inside
It has finished its ride
On its peg it must stay
Till the next day of play.

A Day in the Life of my Coat

A similar poetic approach could be used to encourage children to wear warm coats in cold and wet weather.

A friend for my back
Waits on the coat rack
When I play outside
It comes for a ride!
The cold wind may blow
It can rain or snow
If I go out alone
I get chilled to the bone.
My friend keeps me drier
Like a warm cosy fire.

The Thank-You Princess
by Dawn Tranter

Note from the author: I had worked in a variety of ways to encourage kindergarten children to say 'Thank-you' (but tried to avoid saying to them 'Say thank-you'). Then I wrote this story. After hearing the story the children would play with 'Thank-you' e.g. 'Thank-you lunch box for letting me open you', 'Thank-you drink bottle for holding my drink.' This story offered a playful way of building up the habit of good manners.

In a village, far beyond the hills, where streams trickled over rocks, where birds built their nests in the branches of the many tall trees, there lived a Princess. This Princess was known as the *Thank-you* Princess.

Once upon a time this Princess was happy, oh she was ever so happy, her cheeks glowed with health, her hair shone and her eyes sparkled. What made this little Princess so healthy, so happy? Why, all the times that *Thank-you* was spoken in the world. Every time someone said *Thank-you*, the little Princess's eyes would sparkle just that bit brighter. When a small child said; '*Thank-you* for my dinner', the Princess's hair would grow shiny. When a kind person said; '*Thank-you* ever so much', the Princess's cheeks would have such a rosy glow.

But slowly, so slowly, this little Princess grew pale, this little Princess grew tired. She stopped playing, her eyes lost their sparkle. No longer did her hair grow shiny, no longer did her cheeks have their rosy glow. Why did this little Princess become such an unhappy Princess?

Once upon a time, there were so many *Thank-yous* ringing around the world ... a little boy thanking Daddy for tying his shoe lace, another thanking Mother for cooking such a delicious meal, a girl thanking her friend for helping her build a sandcastle, Father thanking Mother for all the love she brings into the home. So many *Thank-yous* – once upon a time.

But one by one the *Thank-yous* had faded away until the Thank-you Princess found it hard to remember what *Thank-you* even sounded like. She knew only too well all of the 'Do my shoes up, I want a drink, cut my apple' – these she knew only too well.

One night the little Princess's mother visited a house where no *Thank-yous* seemed to live. She had seen a small child that day demanding, 'Make me a sandwich, brush my hair, button my shirt.' All of this the Princess's mother had heard – but not one *Thank-you*.

That same night the Princess's mother took this same small child to visit the Princess's village. The small child saw the beauty of the village, the sparkling streams, the tall trees where the birds built their nests; all of this made the small child feel so happy. But when the small child walked past one of the little cottages and looked in the window, his heart nearly broke. There, sitting in a chair, was the saddest little girl the small child had ever, ever seen. Her eyes were sad, her lips were sad, oh she was so sad. 'Who is this little girl?' cried out the small child, 'why is she so sad?'

'She is my daughter,' the Queen said softly, 'she is known as the *Thank-you* Princess'. 'But why is she so sad?' the small child asked again. 'She grows sadder and paler by the day', said the Queen, 'for there are not enough *Thank-yous* ringing around the world. She used to be so happy, and so healthy. Her eyes would twinkle, her cheeks were rosy, but alas, it seems people no longer think saying *Thank-you* is important. But it is, it is ever so good. For not only does every *Thank-you* go ringing around the world to reach the *Thank-you* Princess, but every *Thank-you* goes straight to the heart of the person we thank. And each time we thank someone our own eyes sparkle a little more.'

The small child was very quiet and very thoughtful as the Queen took him back home.

The next morning, as soon as the small child opened his eyes and looked out the window and saw Father Sun shining so beautifully, he threw open the window and called out in such a happy voice, 'Oh *Thank-you* Father Sun for your beautiful golden sunshine.'

When he dressed and went downstairs his little sister had already set the breakfast table: '*Thank-you* so much for setting the table', he said. And all through the day, without even having to look, the small child found so many things to be thankful for. '*Thank-you* for letting me play, *Thank-you* for being so kind, *Thank-you* for helping me, *Thank-you, Thank-you*'.

The people he thanked found themselves feeling so happy that they soon were thanking people in turn, and very soon there were so many *Thank-you*s ringing around the world that the *Thank-you* Princess slowly began to get better. Her cheeks began to get their old rosy glow back, her hair shone and her beautiful eyes sparkled once again like the stars.

One night, as the small child lay in bed, just before he fell asleep, he heard a faint ringing sound. He listened and could hear, '*Thank-you, Thank-you* ever so much.' The small child's heart felt warm, his cheeks grew rosy, his eyes sparkled, for the *Thank-you* Princess had smiled upon him.

And oh, I shall tell you one more thing, the *Thank-you* Princess has a friend called Prince *Please*, and 'Please' and 'Thank-you' go beautifully together.

Kipury: An African Midwinter Story

I first heard this story from a Kenyan teacher and I have rewritten it to suit children aged five to eight. It is a lovely example of caring and respect, in which a child cares so much for his little lost lamb that he is prepared to risk everything to search for it.

Once upon a time in an African village there lived a young boy named Kipury. Every day the boy woke up with the sun and went out onto the plains herding the sheep while his father was herding the cattle. Just before the sun began to set, he would come back and put the animals safely inside the fence near his hut so no lion could come to steal them.

One day Kipury came back early and put the sheep safely inside the fence. Once he had finished all his work for the day he took his favourite little lamb and walked down to his favourite grove of thorn trees. He sat under the trees, listening to the songs of the birds and watching the little lamb grazing.

After a while Kipury became tired and fell asleep. By that time the little lamb had become thirsty, and since there was no water nearby, it wandered off, searching further and further away.

After quite a while Kipury woke up, rubbed his eyes and looked around. But wherever he looked he could not see the lamb. He then called as loud as he could, but there was no answer. The lamb was nowhere to be seen. And then he went off to search for it ... *(I suggest a song or hum at this point in the story).*

Quite soon he came to a thorny path. Carefully he made his way, and soon he heard a very weak sound. He looked up and saw a bird that was caught in the branches of a thorn bush. 'Cheep cheep', cried the little bird, 'please dear little boy, help me, my wings are caught in the thorns'. 'I cannot help', replied Kipury, 'because I am in a hurry to find my little lamb who is lost.'

Just as he was about to walk on, he thought of his little lamb who also might be in need of help, so he quickly went back. 'Yes little bird, I will help you', said Kipury. The thorns scratched his arms and hands but he carried on until the bird was free. 'Thank-you, thank-you', chirped the bird, filled with joy! ' Now I can fly again! God bless you, and goodbye.' So saying, he flew away.

Kipury went on in search of the lamb ... *(song or hum).*

After a while he came to an open plain where it was hot, dry and dusty. He sat down in a patch of shade, and was taking out his meat to eat and some milk to drink when a little girl came and sat down next to him. 'Dear little boy', she said, 'I have been walking for many days without anything to eat or drink, please have a heart and share what you have with me'. And without hesitating Kipury shared his food with the starving little girl. 'But now I have to hurry because I have to find my lost lamb', said Kipury. 'God bless you', said the little girl, and happily ran away.

Kipury went on with his journey. By that time he was feeling tired, but he still carried on looking for the lamb ... *(song or hum).* Soon he reached a forest. Walking through the shady trees he suddenly heard a noise in front of him and when he looked to see what it was, he saw a big hole in the ground. Trapped inside was a large tortoise. 'You were sent by God', said the tortoise when she saw the boy. 'I have been caught in here a very long time, waiting for someone to help me, and now you have come!' Kipury laid down on the ground, stretched out his arms as far as he could, summoned all of his strength and pulled and pulled the large tortoise out of the trap. You can imagine how grateful the tortoise was to be free again! By this time Kipury felt very tired and hungry, and large tears fell down from his eyes. 'What makes you so sad?', asked the tortoise.

'I have walked so far to find my little lost lamb but to no avail. Now it is getting dark and I don't have any hope of finding it', answered Kipury 'Don't cry,' said the big tortoise, 'Let me help you. Just follow me', and so they walked on together.

As the first stars appeared they reached a dark cave.' Be patient and wait here for a while,' said the tortoise to Kipury, and then she disappeared into the forest. So there Kipury stood, alone in the darkness, not knowing what to do but wait.

All of a sudden he saw a bright light shining out of the cave; and then an old man came forward carrying a shining lantern. 'I have been waiting for you', said the wise old man to the boy. 'The animals have been telling me about you and your good deeds, and now I will help you' and he went into his cave and bought out Kipury's little lamb. The lamb was bleating with joy, and how happy the boy was to have his lamb back! 'Take this lantern,' said the old man, 'and it will guide you safely all the way home'; and so saying he disappeared back into his cave.

Kipury held his light carefully as new strength flowed into him. With his lantern in his hand and his lamb at his side he hurried light-footed all the way home. Kipury's mother saw the light from afar and stretched out her arms to welcome her beloved son home.

The Wombat Family

A 'weaning' story by Kristen Palazzo

The following is an interesting example of how the 'power of story' might help in any situation, even for a mother trying to wean her three-and-a-half-year-old son! When Kristen asked me about this in a workshop in Singapore, I quietly thought to myself, 'I don't know that a story could help wean a child!' I was soon to be proved wrong – as Kristen told me in an email sent a few weeks later. I think it was such an amazing experience for this mother that I have included the full report below. This mother needed to find a way to care for herself as well as her child (she was tired and exhausted when I met her, and in desperate need of help). Her son's favourite toy was a wombat. Since the wombat mother carries her baby in her pouch, this metaphor was a very good choice.

Dear Susan, the story you helped me write had a profound effect on our family's experience during what was a very difficult process. I'd like to share my experience with you. Also I've attached the final version of the story. I had been working on gradually weaning my son Oliver since mid-August (he is 3½ so I felt it was really time). I had a trip planned with two other moms to go to Bangkok for the weekend at the end of September. So my goal was to have finished weaning by the time of my trip, thinking that it would actually help the process if I were not there for a couple of days. The week before my trip I was feeling a little hopeless about being able to wean Oliver by the time of my trip (or at all really) since he was extremely resistant to giving up breast-milk. Thankfully your workshop came at exactly the right moment!

The workshop was on Saturday. I finished the story by the following morning and began telling it that Sunday afternoon. Oliver asked for it about four or five more times that day, and that evening before bed. On Sunday morning we had agreed that Monday morning would be our last wake-up milk. On Monday he asked for the story a bunch more times. Monday night at bed-time I reminded him that the next morning when he woke up, if it was still dark he should try to go back to sleep and when he did call for me I would come in; and if it was late enough we would just get up. I also reminded him about my trip coming up in a few days and said that when we said goodbye for my trip we would also be saying goodbye to 'milky' because now he was ready to graduate from having milk. The next morning when he woke up it was pretty early and still dark. I went into his room and he said he wanted to get up and didn't mention milk at all – usually it's the first thing he says. We debated a bit about getting up and finally we got up, turned on the light and then he asked for the story. So I started to tell the story and we ended up acting out each part of the story – at his prompting. It was really amazing. Then after a while we got up. I think the story really helped us get through the week. He did ask for milk in the morning a few times after that, but at different times he asked some questions related to the story, like 'When baby wombat gets bigger, he doesn't milk any more, right?' So it was clear that the story was having an effect.Anyway, the week went on, I left on Friday, he said goodbye easily and he had a nice weekend with his dad.

When I returned he did want milk to go to sleep and it wasn't an easy few days, but we read the story a bunch more and he asked some questions about what happened to the milk (I told him it had gone back to the moon now that he didn't need it any more, which he didn't like at first). After a few days he was mostly accepting. A big step for us – probably bigger for me than for him! Incidentally, now that he is not asking for milk any more he is not very interested in the story either. I guess it served its purpose – sort of like medicine in a way. It did its healing job and then we put it away.

Once there was a wombat family – a mama wombat, a dada wombat and a baby wombat. Mama wombat carried baby wombat around in her pouch for a very long time until baby wombat was no longer a baby. But baby wombat loved being in his mama's pouch so much that he never wanted to leave! It was very warm and soft and that was where he had his mama's milk.

One day, mama wombat told baby wombat that he was getting too big for her pouch. He was becoming very heavy and it was becoming difficult for mama wombat to walk and to dig. And we all know how much wombats love to dig. After a while he became so heavy that mama wombat could barely move. One day she told baby wombat that very soon it would be time for her to go on a journey. A journey she would have to take alone – she needed to go and find some new special food to make her strong again.

But before she was to go, there was much digging to be done. Mama and dada wombat were planning to dig a bigger home because baby wombat was growing up and needed more space to play and live. So on the digging day, mama and dada wombat began to dig. Baby wombat watched from inside the pouch. Some of the neighbouring wombats heard about the big digging project and came to join them – including their baby wombats. As he watched he started to notice how much fun they were all having. Finally he couldn't stand it any more – he jumped out of the pouch and started to dig himself. He couldn't believe how good it felt. Then he looked down at his feet and suddenly saw what big digging claws he had. He hadn't even realized! This was so exciting! He just kept digging and digging and digging and it felt better than anything else he had ever experienced. He began laughing and singing along with everyone. (Wombats also love to sing especially while they are digging.)

We love digging. Doo-doo-doo doo-doo-doo doo-doo-doo.
We love digging. Doo-doo-doo doo-doo-doo doo-doo-doo.
We love digging. Doo-doo-doo doo-doo-doo doo-doo-doo.
We love digging. Doo-doo-doo doo-doo-doo doo-doo-doo.
(Song sung to the 80s tune 'I love candy')

Once baby wombat was happily digging, mama wombat said it was time for her journey. Baby wombat gave her a big kiss goodbye and then he began to dig next to his dad. They started digging faster and faster – his dad couldn't believe how fast and strong his son was able to dig. They began digging a tunnel. Then from that tunnel they dug another tunnel. Then from that tunnel they dug still another tunnel. They kept digging tunnels until after a while they were right back where they started and had dug a whole big maze of tunnels to play in.

Not long after they finished their tunnels, mama wombat returned from her journey. Mama wombat was so happy to see that her baby had become strong and big. Baby wombat was so excited to tell her of all the adventures and fun that he and his dad had had while she was away. Taking her by the hand baby wombat showed her all the tunnels they had built. The new tunnels were now his own warm and soft place.

The Bowing Tree

I have adapted this story from a traditional African fairytale. It has a strong message that greed doesn't pay, and the importance of caring for others. It is suitable for children aged from five to ten.

There was once a village suffering a very long time of famine. The grains in the fields and the vegetables in the garden had all died from lack of water, and the food that had been stored in the grain bins was slowly running out. Every day each family only had a small handful of rice and beans to cook up in their pot and share around. Every evening all the families would meet in the village square to pray together for rain.

But there was one man in the village who was not suffering from lack of food. This was the village chief. He had gone walking one day far from home to look for water and had found an old giant tree growing by the edge of a dusty riverbed. The chief sat down to rest in the shade of the tree, and while he was sitting there he began to sing of the famine in his village. All of a sudden his song was interrupted by a groaning and creaking, and to the chief's surprise, he watched as the tree bowed down all of its great branches and delivered many fruits to the ground below. The chief quickly gathered them up and sat feasting on the delicious fruits as the tree lifted its branches back up towards the sky.

The chief, with his belly now fully satisfied, set off to walk the long distance home. When he arrived, his wife was about to serve up the small portion of rice and beans to his family. Thinking her husband would be hungry after his long walk, she served extra food for him, but he refused, saying 'Give it to the children – they must eat. I will go hungry tonight.' Then the chief went to bed, leaving his wife full of admiration for her selfless husband who was prepared to go hungry so his children would not starve.

The following day, the chief made his way to the dry riverbed, sat under the giant tree and sang a song of the famine, just as before. And just as before, his song was interrupted by a groaning and creaking, and he watched as the tree bowed down all of its great branches and delivered many fruits to the ground below. The chief quickly gathered them up and sat feasting on the delicious fruits as the tree lifted its branches back up towards the sky.

At home that evening, the chief once again declined the offer of food from his wife, saying 'I cannot eat until my children are fat once more.' Then he went to bed, leaving his wife even more astonished at her husband's goodness … a man who was prepared to go hungry so his children would not starve!

This continued for many days. The chief would walk each day to the great tree and after singing to the tree he would feast on its wonderful fruits. Then he would return home and refuse to eat any food offered by his wife, saying he would prefer that she give it to his children. Soon all of the villagers had heard about this selfless behaviour and felt in awe of the goodness of their chief.

Now it is possible that life could have continued in this way for longer than many days … many months perhaps … except for one thing. One of the chief's young sons had grown very curious as to how his father had not eaten for so long, but was growing fatter and fatter by the day. So this boy decided to follow him one morning on his walk to the dusty riverbed. The boy hid behind a rock and watched as his father sat down in the shade of the great tree. The boy listened as his father sang his song of the famine and then watched in great surprise as the tree bowed down all its branches and gave delicious fruits to eat.

Quickly and quietly the boy ran back to the village and told his mother all that he had seen. The mother was distraught with anger when she heard of the greedy behaviour of her husband. She then thought of a plan to teach her husband a good lesson.

Early the next morning, when her husband had left for his walk, the mother gathered up all her children and led them quietly along the path to the dusty riverbed. The chief did not know that his family was following him. As he reached the giant tree, his wife and children ran up, stood under the branches, and sang out loudly:

A selfish man likes to fill his belly while his family wait at home with little food to share.

On hearing this song, the tree made a huge groaning and shuddering and creaking, much louder than ever before, and then its giant branches bent to the ground offering fruits of all kinds and shapes and flavours to the children and the chief's wife.

The chief was very ashamed to be caught out like this, and tried to pretend that he had just discovered the magic of the tree. 'This tree has food for all of us' he cried out. But when he bent down to pick a fruit and put it in his mouth, it tasted so bitter he had to spit it straight back out. He tried another fruit and another, but everyone he tried was like bitter poison in his mouth. Meanwhile his wife and children feasted as they never had before, and all the fruit they tasted was sweet and wonderful.

The next day the wife led all the villagers back to the giant tree. They carried baskets and pots and they stood under the tree and sang a wonderful song. The tree bowed down its great branches laden with fruits and the villagers filled their baskets and pots to overflowing with the wonderful food. That night back in the village, a great feast was held to celebrate how the fruits from the magic tree had ended the famine.

But the chief, who no longer could taste such wonderful food without it being like bitter poison in his mouth, went to bed after only a small bowl of rice and beans to eat.

The Ocean Playground

Chengdu teacher training, China. This story idea was aimed at a class of five-year-old children who weren't caring for their toys – in particular there was one boy who was clumsy and broke things and knocked things over.

Once upon a time many sea creatures lived at the bottom of the deep blue sea. There was Crab, Shrimp and Seahorse, and they all liked to play together in their sea garden. Each day they would use shells and stones to build houses, then they played hide-and-seek in and around the houses.

One day Octopus came to visit for the first time. The sea creatures welcomed this new arrival but when they began to build houses together the long tentacles of the octopus kept breaking the walls down.

After this happened many times, Crab, Shrimp and Seahorse decided to move to a new playground, away from this visitor who kept breaking their houses down. Octopus tried to follow them but his many tentacles kept knocking more things over. He bumped into so many things that his tentacles were covered in broken pieces of shell and stone. Soon he was trapped under the mess. He called out for help but no one heard. The other sea creatures were too busy playing in their new playground.

Finally Octopus managed to wriggle one of his tentacles backwards and forwards. This wriggling movement attracted a little fish. The little fish quickly saw what had happened to poor Octopus and swam off to get the others. Crab, Shrimp and Seahorse returned to help lift all the bits and pieces off Octopus's back.

Once he was free, Octopus realized that if he moved very slowly and carefully he could stop breaking and knocking things. He soon became good friends with the other sea creatures and they loved playing with him, as he had so many hands to help with building!

'Story bones' – The Golden Feather

Sydney: this story idea was suggested for a six-year-old who often took other children's things without asking. It highlights the joy of returning things, and having respect and care for property that belongs to others.

Story about a magic bird with a golden feather. This bird loves to dance high in the sky – down below a magpie watches the golden feather glinting in the sunlight – and wishes it could have a golden feather too. One day while the magic bird is dancing it drops its golden feather. A magpie finds it and flies up high, trying to dance with it. It puts it into one wing, but it won't stay there; it puts it into the other wing, but the feather won't stay in place; then it tries to put it into a headband but no matter what the magpie does, the golden feather doesn't seem to help it dance like the magic bird.

Eventually the magpie flies out to find the magic bird and gives it back its golden feather. The magic bird is so happy to have its special feather back. It tucks it back into its wings, and then it offers to teach the magpie a special dance. The two birds dance together in the sky for the rest of the day.

8

Disruptive/Restless/Over-excited

Juju Finds a Friend

A story for fidgety, restless children

The idea for this story about Juju came from observing my kindergarten children one day. A group of the five-year-olds were playing near an old house at the edge of the park, and I watched as one, then another, then the whole group, stood quietly at the hedge peering though at something. I was amazed at how long they all stood still, and eventually I joined them. They were watching a stone statue of a little Indian prince. It was in the middle of an overgrown garden and the children were keeping quiet and very still as they thought it was a real boy. They were waiting for it to move! The next day we returned to the park so the children could see if the boy was still there. Then it started to rain and we left quickly, but the children were concerned that the little boy would get wet, and one child wanted to take an umbrella back to keep the statue dry.

There was once a little girl who could never keep still. Her father called her Juju and even her name had a jump in its sound.

Juju jumped around from the moment she woke in the morning till the moment she fell asleep at night. She jumped around the house, she jumped over the garden beds, she skipped and jumped along the forest path, she ran and jumped all through the park. If it hadn't been for her seatbelt, Juju would have liked to jump up and down on the car seat when her father was driving her to town!

Sometimes her father would sigh, 'I wish you could sometimes be still as a stone.'

But Juju was not a stone and Juju didn't want to keep still. 'I like to move and jump around' she would tell her father, 'that's what little children do. Stones like to keep still, children like to move.'

(The truth is that Juju wouldn't have known how to keep still, even if she had wanted to try!)

Every afternoon after work, her father would take her to the park so that Juju had time and space to run and jump around. Father would always have his rug and book with him, in case he had a chance to read a page or two! While he rested, Juju climbed and jumped out of the trees, hopped and jumped over the stones and logs, and ran backwards and forwards across the little bridge over the creek.

One day, Juju and her father visited a different corner of the park. This took them near an old house with a hedged garden that Juju had never seen before. While her father spread out his rug on the grass and lay down to try and read his book, Juju ran up to the hedge at the edge of the garden and peered through the leaves.

She was very surprised at what she saw.

In the middle of the garden, standing inside a round bed of flowers, was a little boy just about her size.

'Hello', whispered Juju, 'do you want to be my friend?' But the stone boy didn't answer. Juju stood watching him for a minute, wondering why her new friend wouldn't reply. Then she returned to play in the park, but after a few hops and jumps, she was back at the hedge to see if her new friend was still there. And every time she looked, her friend was standing in the same place – he had not moved at all!

That night Juju fell asleep thinking about her new friend.

'Can we go to the new corner of the park today?' Juju asked her father the next afternoon. 'Of course', said her father, who was very pleased at how happily Juju had played the day before and how much of his book he had managed to read!

When they reached the corner of the park near the old house and garden, Juju's father spread out his rug and lay down. Before he started to read he watched Juju for a while. He was surprised to see his little girl standing still near the edge of the garden, peering through the leaves of the hedge. She stood there for an unusually long time, almost two minutes! Then she ran off and hopped in and out the palm trees and climbed a rock pile. But soon she was back, standing still at the edge of the garden and looking through the hedge.

Her father kept reading his book. Today he didn't have to look out for Juju as much as he was used to doing – she just kept returning to the edge of the garden, and standing still. 'She must have found a grasshopper or a beetle to look at', he thought to himself, and decided that from now on they would come to this corner of the park more often.

The next day it was lightly raining and Juju's father wasn't so keen to go walking. But Juju insisted! She also insisted that she take two umbrellas, holding one over her head and holding one, still folded up, in her free hand. 'Children are strange sometimes', thought her father, who usually had a difficult time getting Juju to carry even one umbrella!

When they reached the park, Juju ran straight towards the old garden. As it was too wet to sit on the grass, her father followed her and sat on the remains of the old brick wall near the hedge. He peered through the branches as his little girl carefully and quietly crept through the wet leaves and made her way across the garden. Then he saw the statue! He kept peering through the bushes, watching in amazement.

Juju reached the flower garden where her stone friend lived, and put down her folded umbrella on the wet grass. 'Hello' said Juju to her friend, 'I have brought you an umbrella to keep you from getting too wet and cold.' Juju reached across the flowerbed and placed the handle of the open umbrella in the stone fingers of the boy's hand. Then she propped the canopy of the umbrella over the stone boy's head. When this was done, she stood up, put up her other umbrella and held it over her own head. Holding her umbrella up high, Juju then stood and chatted to her friend for what seemed, to her father, like a very long time!

All this while the rain continued to fall, lightly pitter-pattering down on the garden and the umbrellas. And without Juju knowing, her father continued to watch her from afar.

They didn't stay long at the park that day. When Juju emerged from the bushes to find her father sitting on the wall, it was starting to rain much more heavily than before and Juju seemed content to return home.

Her father never asked her about the second umbrella, and Juju was very happy to keep the *secret* about her new friend to herself.

Juju's father was also very happy – Juju's new friend had helped her to sometimes be 'as still as stone'.

The Three Pots

A Bagandan story told to students at a teacher-training module in Nairobi by Catherine Kabonge from Uganda (transcribed and adapted by Susan Perrow). This story beautifully highlights the importance of staying concentrated on the task at hand. Like many traditional tales, it is not a story just for children. An adult friend of mine who heard this story commented that it seemed to be written just for her – it gave her the strength to pull out of a relationship commitment since the story helped her realize that her partner was not able to stay 'on the path and carry the pot home'. He was too often distracted by beautiful birds!

There was once a woman who lived with her only daughter. The daughter was the kindest, most generous and most beautiful girl in the village, and there were many young men who wished to be her husband.

Her mother wanted to help find the best possible man for her daughter, one who knew how to work hard, stay loyal to his promises, and treat his wife with love and respect. So the mother worked out a test, and announced to the interested men that the one who was able to pass the test would be the one who could marry her daughter.

On the morning of the marrying test there were many men waiting outside the mother's hut.

The first man set off to attempt his task. He was given a clay pot to take to the well and fill with water, and was told he would pass the test if he could return the pot of water unbroken to the hut. He set off, and, on reaching the well, he lowered the pot to fill it with water. Then he put the pot on his shoulder and turned to follow the path back to the mother's hut. As he passed under the shady tree by the well, a golden bird began to sing a glorious song.

Listen to me, listen only to me … I am a golden bird, O listen to me.

The man stopped and turned to listen to the bird, and the pot fell from his shoulder and crashed to the ground. He had failed the test.

The second man set off to attempt his task. He was given a clay pot to take to the well and fill with water, and was told he would pass the test if he could return the pot of water unbroken to the hut. He set off, and, on reaching the well, he lowered the pot to fill it with water. Then he put the pot on his shoulder and turned to follow the path back to the mother's hut. As he passed under the shady tree by the well, a golden bird began to sing a glorious song.

Listen to me, listen only to me … I am a golden bird, O listen to me.

The man stopped and turned to listen to the bird, and the pot fell from his shoulder and crashed to the ground. He had failed the test.

The third man set off to attempt his task. He was given a clay pot to take to the well and fill with water, and was told he would pass the test if he could return the pot of water unbroken to the hut. He set off, and, on reaching the well, he lowered the pot to fill it with water.

Then he put the pot on his shoulder and turned to follow the path back to the mother's hut. As he passed under the shady tree by the well, a golden bird began to sing a glorious song.

Listen to me, listen only to me … I am a golden bird, O listen to me.

The man listened to the bird as he kept on walking. He did not stop and he did not turn around. He continued along the path ahead of him. The pot of water stayed balanced on his shoulder.

When he reached the hut he lifted the pot down and gave it to the mother. The mother called her daughter to the door of the hut. She was very happy to meet the man who could pass such a difficult test. The daughter agreed to take this man as her husband, and that night there was great celebration and feasting in the village.

The golden bird flew from the tree by the well to rest in a tree near the marriage hut, and at dawn, on the day after the wedding, it sang a love song for the newly-wed couple.

Panya the Rat

Panya the Rat was written using African animals and Kiswahili names. It has a similar theme to 'Nibbler the Mouse', a classic Russian nonsense tale about a little mouse who finds an upside-down pot and moves inside it to make it his house. In this version, Panya the Rat finds an old hat lying in the grass, and makes it his dwelling. It is a wonderful story to tell to restless children who struggle to focus at story time – the storyteller can use the five fingers of one hand (to represent the five animals) and an old red hat in the other hand (or a half-closed fist can represent a hat). The children easily become engaged by using their own fingers and hands as puppets. I usually call on a child to come up at the end to make a fist for 'Hyena Squash-the-Lot'.

One day Panya the Rat is wandering across the plains of Africa looking for a new place to make his home. He finds an old red hat lying in the grass, scampers up to it and looks inside.

Little hat, little hat, who lives in this little hat?

Nobody answers, so Panya the Rat goes inside to live in the old red hat.

By and by, through the grass, along comes Chura the Frog. He comes up to the hat and says:

Little hat, little hat, who lives in this little hat?
I do, says Panya the Rat, who are you?
I'm Chura the Frog, may I come and live with you?

So Chura the Frog goes into the old red hat and lives with Panya the Rat.

By and by, through the grass, along comes Sungura the Hare. He comes up to the old red hat and says:

Little hat, little hat, who lives in this little hat?
I do, says Panya the Rat, I do says Chura the Frog, who are you?
I'm Sungura the Hare, may I come and live with you?

So Sungura the Hare goes into the old red hat and lives with Chura the Frog and Panya the Rat.

By and by, through the grass, along comes Tumbili the Monkey. He comes up to the old red hat and says:

Little hat, little hat, who lives in this little hat?
I do, says Panya the Rat, I do says Chura the Frog, I do says Sungura the Hare, who are you?
I'm Tumbili the Monkey, may I come and live with you?

So Tumbili the Monkey goes into the old red hat and lives with Sungura the Hare, Chura the Frog and Panya the Rat.

By and by, through the grass, along comes Swara the Antelope. He comes up to the old red hat and says:

Little hat, little hat, who lives in this little hat?
I do, says Panya the Rat, I do says Chura the Frog, I do says Sungura the Hare, I do says Tumbili the Monkey, who are you?
I'm Swara the Antelope, may I come and live with you?

So Swara the Antelope goes into the old red hat and lives with Tumbili the Monkey, Sungura the Hare, Chura the Frog and Panya the Rat.

By and by, through the grass, along comes Fisi the Hyena. He comes up to the old red hat and says:

Little hat, little hat, who lives in this little hat?
I do, says Panya the Rat, I do says Chura the Frog, I do says Sungura the Hare, I do says Tumbili the Monkey, I do says Swara the Antelope, who are you?

I'm Hyena Squash-the-Lot, says Fisi the Hyena (with a loud hyena laugh – whoop whoop whoop), and he sat on top of the old red hat and tried to squash the lot.

But luckily there was a hole in the side of the old red hat, and just in time all the friends managed to squeeze out. They ran off into the grass to search for new homes, leaving Fisi the Hyena sitting on top of an empty red hat!

The Three Ponies
by Sue Hurst

I wrote this story because I had two girls in my kindergarten group who found it very hard to listen at story time. I felt that this was making it difficult for the other children who really wanted to hear the story. I tried changing the timing of the story, removing some of the children, and other things, with limited success. After reading your book on Healing Stories, *I sat down and wrote The Three Ponies. I told the story for a couple of weeks and, lo and behold, I noticed a change in their behaviour. For the better! They both seemed to be more settled during the telling of stories and now they are six they are both wonderful storytellers themselves.*

Once upon a time there was a herd of wild horses who lived on the mountain plains. Every day they roamed around the tussocks until tired and thirsty, then they would go to drink from the clear mountain pond.

One day they were joined at the water's edge by three little ponies. The horses moved to make room for the ponies to drink their fill – but after drinking a little water the ponies began to jump about in the pond. At first the horses laughed to see the ponies enjoying themselves so much. But then they noticed that the pond was getting muddy and murky. In fact, so muddy and murky that they could no longer drink from it!

Every day when the horses came to the pond the same thing would happen. The horses began to get annoyed that they could no longer enjoy the cool clear water. So they set off to find the wise old donkey who lived nearby, and they asked him what they should do about the ponies muddying the pond.

The wise old donkey said they should go and call to the wide-mouthed frog who lived at the bottom of the pond. He said that the frog had such a wide mouth that he could drink up all the water in the pond and hold it there. 'How will that help?' asked one of the horses. 'Well' answered the wise old donkey 'when the ponies come down there will be no water there for them to drink and play in. 'But', asked the horse 'won't we die of thirst?' 'Ah' said the donkey, 'you must be sure to go down early in the morning to have a drink, when the ponies are not around.'

So the horses went back to the pond and called up the wide-mouthed frog and told him the donkey's plan. The frog said that he did not like the pond being so murky either and agreed to help them. Every morning the horses would go down to drink, and then the frog would take up all the water into his mouth. So when the ponies came to drink and play they found the pond completely dry. After dashing around in the dust the ponies grew tired and thirsty.

Finally, on the third day the ponies came to the horses and said 'We are so thirsty, we haven't had a drink for three whole days – oh how we wish that the cool clear waters of the mountain pool would return.' The horses took pity on them and asked the frog to let go the water and fill the pond back up.

When the ponies came the next day they could drink deeply and satisfy their thirst. They found that they enjoyed the sweet taste of the water so much that they never again jumped around and made it muddy and murky. And from that day onwards the ponies and the horses played together amongst the tussocks and drank together afterwards in the cool, clear waters of the mountain pond.

Mindy at the Country Fair

A soothing story for restless and excited children, with an exciting thread through being presented in a rhythmical, repetitive way. It includes the idea of a dancing stick – can simply be made with a stick and ribbons – that children delight in playing with. Suitable for children aged 4 to 8.

Mindy lived in a little house with her mother on the far side of town. Most of the year, when she was not at school, Mindy loved to play with her friends in the Knocking-Door-Tree Forest at the bottom of her garden. Most of all she loved to dance in and out of the sunbeams that shone down through the dark green leaves and onto the forest path.

But this month was different. It was springtime and many spring-cleaning jobs needed to get done. And so Mindy had been using all her spare time to help her mother. She had been sweeping and dusting in out-of-the-way places, washing windows and walls, and cleaning cupboards that had not been looked in for a year or more.

Finally the jobs were done and it was Sunday. Not just any Sunday! It was 'Country Fair' Sunday and Mindy's mother had given her a golden dollar to spend. The golden dollar was safely tucked into a little bag that hung off a string of pink leather around Mindy's neck. And Mindy was on her way to the fair with one hand holding onto her mother and the other swinging free.

Mindy had a skip in her step and a song for her skip:

A golden treasure has come my way, a golden treasure to spend today!

When they arrived there were people everywhere. Mindy could see the coloured flags flying from the stalls, and she could hear the music from the stage in the middle of the fairground. As she and her mother passed through the gate she could smell the popcorn cooking at the popcorn stall just near the entrance.

'Now Mindy,' said her Mother, 'I have to work on the school stall for a while and then we will watch the grand parade together. You will have to find something to do until I am finished.' Mindy smiled and felt in her purse to see the golden dollar was still safely inside. She knew exactly what she wanted to do.

She skipped past the popcorn stall.

She skipped past the craft stall.

She skipped past the school stall, where she could see her mother busily setting out drinks and food.

And as she skipped, she sang to herself:

A golden treasure has come my way, a golden treasure to spend today!

Mindy knew exactly where she wanted to go.

She skipped past the cake stall,

She skipped past the toy stall,

She skipped past the bookstall, all the while singing to herself:

A golden treasure has come my way, a golden treasure to spend today!

Mindy knew exactly what she wanted to do and Mindy knew exactly where she wanted to go. She remembered from last year what she and her friends had liked the best at the whole fair – and there it was, she could see it now, set out on a large white net under the trees – *the Magic Fishing Dip!*

Already some children were lining up to take their turn to catch a coloured wool fish, and then collect a matching-colour prize from the prize basket. Mindy joined the line, still happily singing:

A golden treasure has come my way, a golden treasure to spend today!

As the line moved along, Mindy was able to see the coloured fish scattered in the net amongst the shells and seaweed – blue fish, red fish, yellow fish, green fish, orange fish and pink fish. And right at the back of the net, Mindy could see one large purple fish.

In the prize basket next to the net, there was one long box wrapped in purple paper sticking out above all the rest. 'That's the one for me', she thought.

Finally it was Mindy's turn! She took her golden dollar out of her purse and handed it to the Fishing Dip man, and the man gave Mindy a bamboo fishing rod. The rod had a prickly seedpod hook on the end of a piece of string. 'Three turns only', he said.

Mindy stepped up to the front of the line and had her first try, throwing out her prickly hook into the net. But when she pulled it back in, there was nothing there!

On her second go, all she managed to catch was a curly piece of seaweed! 'Last try' said the Fishing Dip man.

Mindy closed her eyes and made a wish. With her eyes still closed, she threw out her hook as far as she could. Then she heard the children behind her cheer and shout, and when she opened her eyes, there, caught fast in the prickles of her fishing hook, was the large purple fish!

'Well done', said the Fishing Dip man. 'That was such a good catch … maybe you should take up *real* fishing'. And he handed Mindy the long purple prize from the basket.

'*Magic* fishing is much better', thought Mindy to herself as she thanked the man. She was so excited that her fingers could hardly open the box, but when she finally managed to open one end and reach inside, what do you think she found?

Exactly what she had wished for – a rainbow ribbon stick! Mindy was so happy. She skipped and danced with the ribbon stick back to the school stall to show her mother, singing all the way:

> *A rainbow treasure has come my way, a rainbow treasure to dance with today!*

At the end of the day, after the grand parade, and after eating a fruit salad ice-block and a large bag of popcorn, Mindy took hold of her mother's hand and set out for home. In her other hand she was tightly holding her special prize. Together they walked the long road across town, with Mindy chatting all the way about the Magic Fishing Dip.

As soon as she reached her garden she ran straight to where the forest path led under the shady trees. Although it was late in the afternoon some sunlight was still shining down onto the leafy path. Mindy held her ribbon stick up high and started to dance, weaving the rainbow colours in and out of the golden sunbeams.

Mindy had never felt so happy! What a joy it was to dance like this, in and out of the golden shafts of light.

And for all I know, she may still be dancing there today, with a skip in her step and a song for her skip. So if you go walking through the Knocking-Door-Tree Forest, you may meet a little girl with a rainbow ribbon stick, dancing and singing to herself:

> *a a a a a a b g a*
> *A rainbow treasure has come my way,*
> *a a a a a a   g g b a*
> *A rainbow treasure to dance with today.*

Note to the children: You can make your own ribbon stick by tying short lengths of coloured ribbon or wool on the end of a stick (the stick needs to be strong, straight and smooth, and about as long as from your fingertips to your elbow). Then you can take it to the forest and dance in and out of the golden sunbeams.

Wombat Helps to Build a Dam

At a workshop on the South Coast of NSW, a group of teachers came up with a mixture of 'story bones' and some rhyming lines for a five-year-old girl who overreacts to situations then feels helpless, upset and powerless to change things. The story (completed below) aimed to encourage her to 'take part in solutions' instead of overreacting and getting distressed.

There was once a mother wombat and a baby wombat out walking along a bush path. The path led them to a dam. It had been raining and the dam was full to the top. Suddenly the dam wall cracked on one side and the water came flooding through the crack.

The baby wombat ran off into the bush land, crying out for help. He met a platypus and the platypus asked,

> *Why the hurry, why the worry, for one so small?*

The baby wombat replied:

> *There is a crack in the dam wall and I feel too small to fix it all,*
> *The water's coming through and I don't know what to do!*

The baby wombat kept running through the bush land, crying out for help.

He met a kangaroo and the kangaroo asked,

Why the hurry, why the worry, for one so small?

The baby wombat replied:

There is a crack in the dam wall and I feel too small to fix it all,
The water's coming through and I don't know what to do!

The baby wombat kept running through the bush land, crying out for help.

He met a koala and the koala asked,

Why the hurry, why the worry, for one so small?

The baby wombat replied:

There is a crack in the dam wall and I feel too small to fix it all,
The water's coming through and I don't know what to do!

The baby wombat kept running through the bush land, crying out for help.

He met a kookaburra and the kookaburra asked,

Why the hurry, why the worry, for one so small?

The baby wombat replied:

There is a crack in the dam wall and I feel too small to fix it all,
The water's coming through and I don't know what to do!

The baby wombat eventually ran full circle through the bush land and arrived back at the dam. To her surprise she found all her friends busy fixing the wall – the platypus, the kangaroo, the koala, the kookaburra and mother wombat.

Mother wombat was so happy to see her baby return safely. She called out,

Let us all give out a cheer, our wombat helper is here.

Baby wombat realized that by meeting all those friends on the path she had found a way to get them all involved. Baby wombat snuggled up to her mother and happily replied,

I wasn't too small to find a way to fix it all!

The Frangipani Gift

A soothing summer Christmas story for four- to six-year-olds about patiently waiting and taking time!

All through the long springtime, the flower children were dancing in the garden. Daisies, jasmine, pansies and marigolds – all with their coloured dresses shining in the bright spring light.

But there was one flower child who had not come out to dance. Frangipani was still sleeping, deep in the branches of her frangipani tree.

Every day the flower children would dance around the brown bare branches of the frangipani tree, calling:

Frangipani Child – come out, come out, to dance and play,
Springtime is here and the world is bright and gay.

But still the Frangipani Child kept sleeping, and the wind would whisper to the flower children:

Frangipani is waiting for a special time,
Frangipani is waiting for a golden light to shine.

Every day the bees would buzz around the brown bare branches of the frangipani tree, calling:

Frangipani Child – come out, come out, to dance and play,
Springtime is here and the world is bright and gay.

But still the Frangipani Child kept sleeping, and the wind would whisper to the busy buzzing bees:

Frangipani is waiting for a special time,
Frangipani is waiting for a golden light to shine

Every day the butterflies would flutter around the brown bare branches of the frangipani tree, calling:

Frangipani Child – come out, come out, to dance and play,
Springtime is here and the world is bright and gay.

But still the Frangipani Child kept sleeping, and the wind would whisper to the fluttering butterflies:

Frangipani is waiting for a special time,
Frangipani is waiting for a golden light to shine

Summer came to the garden, and now the frangipani tree wore a soft green dress. The flower children kept calling to the Frangipani Child, the busy bees kept calling to the Frangipani Child, the fluttering butterflies kept calling to the Frangipani Child, but still she kept sleeping … and the wind whispered:

Frangipani is waiting for a special time,
Frangipani is waiting for a golden light to shine

Finally that special time came, the time of Christmas, when the Child of Light came walking in the summer garden. As the Child of Light passed the frangipani tree, the Frangipani Child woke up, stretched out her white petal arms, and offered her gift of beautiful perfume. And as the Child of Light reached up to smell the beautiful perfume, a shining golden light seemed to 'kiss' the Frangipani Child and her heart began to shine in a wonderful golden glow.

And from that day to this, the Frangipani Child has always had a glowing golden heart, and always gives her gift of perfume to the world at summer, around Christmas time.

'Story bones' – The Ants' Feast

At a workshop in Sydney this story idea was shared by a mother for her four-and-a-half-year-old who gets over-excited and disruptive before special events.

The story is about a busy colony of ants – preparing for a feast – an ant tunnel leads into an amphitheatre where the feast will be held – on the day before the feast the ants were rushing round so fast that many ants got stuck in the tunnel – the ants ended up so squashed together that they couldn't go forwards or backwards – then one ant sat down and started to hum a song – all the ants followed this example and they all sat down and sang together. Slowly the ants started to move out of the tunnel in a slow and rhythmical pace, singing about what jobs they had to do. The preparations happened in a calm way and the feast was a great success for all involved.

9

Dishonest/Sneaky

Juniper the Rabbit
by Didi A. Devapriya

Didi contacted me from her AMURTEL project in Romania, where she was supervising a small foster-care children's home. She explained that she faced particularly challenging forms of behaviour as these kids were traumatized by extremely neglectful care in their earliest years after being abandoned by their birth parents. Didi wrote the story below to help the children (and staff) have a more compassionate and insightful understanding of the challenging behaviour. She reported that she had twice told it in Romanian to the children. In her words: 'They were really fascinated, connected and giggling during the telling and they were definitely identifying with the character. White rabbits were a current favourite pet (we even have one called "Juniper") so that is why I picked that animal, and the next day one of them came to me to show me "Juniper" ... he also re-told the whole story for me quite accurately. I feel that the story helped the children to connect and engage, and not feel so isolated in their trauma and behaviour.'

Juniper was a white baby rabbit. She lived with twenty-seven other baby rabbits inside a small cage. It was very crowded and uncomfortable. When the farmer came with food, all of the rabbits scrambled on top of each other, fighting for their share.

Juniper was small and not very fast, and the others climbed over her and ate up most of the food before her. She was always still hungry when the food was finished, and cried for more, but nobody listened. They were too busy trying to get food for themselves.

One day, a little boy came and chose five rabbits to take home as pets. Juniper was small and white and very shy, and the boy liked her. The five little rabbits had a bumpy ride inside a straw basket. The loud sounds of a car motor were frightening and there were so many new smells; and light was flickering through the weave of the straw basket. They didn't know what was happening, and the scared baby rabbits huddled together, shivering with fear.

At last, when the basket was opened, Juniper was lifted up and found herself in a new home. This one was big and roomy, with lots of soft straw, and two big green ceramic bowls. One was full of food and the other with water. The rabbits scrambled hungrily to the food dishes, especially Juniper. She pushed her way through the other rabbits and gathered up as much food as she could carry in her paws; then went to a corner of the cage to eat and eat as much as she could. Still she was hungry – but there was more, and again she took it away from the others so that they wouldn't eat it first. Even after many days, and nights Juniper was still always scared that there wouldn't be enough food for her. She never wanted to feel hungry again, so she always took her food and ate quickly by herself, as much as she could, even when she wasn't really hungry.

The boy liked to play with the rabbits, picking them up and petting them and giving them food from his hand. But Juniper was scared when the boy came to pick her up; and she would run to her safe corner of the cage where her bed was. Sometimes she felt bad that the other rabbits got extra food and attention from the boy. When he wasn't looking she would bite them or scratch them. They were afraid of her, and avoided her, so she spent a lot of time feeling lonely and sad and that nobody cared about her.

One day the boy came to the cage and said, 'Look what I have!' to the little rabbits. He was holding up a jar of carrot and cabbage salad that he had saved from his dinner. The rabbits were very excited, sniffing the scent of sweet carrot and juicy cabbage leaves. It was their favourite dessert! The boy promised them a special treat in the morning for breakfast.

That night when everyone was sleeping, Juniper woke up. She was really excited about the carrot salad. But when she thought about it, she was also afraid there wouldn't be enough for her. She was a clever rabbit: she looked carefully at the latch that kept her cage shut, and discovered a way to open it with her teeth. Then she crept quietly, quietly out of the cage. She found the jar of salad, and began munching hungrily. She ate and ate, until she was very, very full. Then she took as much as she could carry in her paws and hid it under her straw pillow, so she could eat more later. She closed the door carefully and then went to sleep.

When the boy woke up in the morning, he looked for the jar of salad to give to his rabbits. He found it toppled over and almost finished. He was very angry that someone had ruined the treat he had planned for the rabbits and started to shout, 'Somebody took the salad! Who could it be?' The rabbits had never seen the boy angry, and it made them all very scared, especially Juniper – who ran to her bed and sat on her pillow. Her heart was beating very fast, her paws trembled and she felt cold and shivery. Then the boy came to the rabbits, looking very sad and disappointed. 'I am really sorry bunnies – somebody ate up all of your salad, and there is no more … ' The little bunnies were very disappointed too. They had really been looking forward to their treat.

That night, when finally everyone was sleeping, Juniper brushed aside the straw to find her buried carrot salad treasure … She started nibbling on it – she knew she had to finish it quickly or the others might discover what she had done and be angry. But somehow, it didn't taste quite as sweet as the night before … and her heart was beating fast, and she felt uncomfortable.

Wise spider on the wall called out to her, 'Juniper, I see that it was you who took the salad.' Juniper jumped with fright, her heart pounding. 'What salad? Of course I didn't take it – I just found it. I mean, someone else must have taken it and hid it here', she said in a shaky voice. Wise spider said, 'Hmmm … . Juniper, you don't need to be frightened – I am not going to hurt you, and you are not in trouble. I am just a small spider, but I know many things. I understand that you were the smallest and had to fight to get your food when you were very little, and even now you are not sure that the boy will give you enough to eat. But, you know, he is good and he really does want to be your friend. I think you can trust him. He would love to pick you up and feed you sweet salad leaves from his hand like the others; you just need to let him get close to you.'

Juniper thought about that. She also thought about the other bunnies, and how sad and disappointed they had been that the salad was gone. 'What am I going to do with this salad now?' she said to the spider, feeling very sad and ashamed. The spider came close and whispered a secret in her long bunny ear. Juniper smiled.

The next morning, each bunny woke up to find a cabbage leaf full of carrot salad right next to their nose. The bunnies were very happy and excited and called to the boy. He was also surprised and happy. He came to pick them up and pet them. He saw Juniper didn't have a leaf of salad like the others and so he picked her up to give her some special food from his hand. Juniper took a big deep breath when he came to pick her up to wash away the fear building up in her … and then suddenly she was in his arms and it felt warm and snuggly. As Juniper ate the lettuce in his hand, the boy told her 'You know, a wise spider came and told me a secret.' Juniper's heart froze … and she started to tremble. Was he going to be angry?

He said, 'I know you took the salad, and that you took it because you are afraid you won't get enough. I promise you I will always take special care to make sure you have enough to eat, and I will also feed you specially from my hand.'

Juniper was so relieved that he wasn't angry, and that he under-stood her and wanted to be her friend. She snuggled in his arms and felt very warm and happy inside. She and the boy became very, very good friends and she always had enough to eat, so she never had to take food and hide it from the others again.

Forest Boy and the Red Shoes

A story written for five-year-olds as a gentle approach to a 'stealing' situ-ation in a group of friends – concentrating more on helping rectify the situation and less on the act of stealing. It was performed as a puppet show, with the involvement of all the friends. They were all enchanted by the storyline and took the message into their creative play – hiding things then finding them again. This helped address the stealing behaviour.

Forest Boy lived in a hollow tree in the middle of the bush. He had a soft bed of leaves to sleep on, lots of berries and nuts to eat, and many friends to play with. He was very happy with his life.

One of Forest Boy's favourite things was his red shoes. They were soft and warm for his feet, and they helped him move quietly on the forest paths, especially when he didn't want goanna or snake to know he was passing by their homes!

Forest Boy wore his red shoes everywhere … except to bed of course! At night he would take them off and leave them just inside his door, ready to put on when he woke each morning.

But one night, while Forest Boy was sleeping, something came and took one of his red shoes. In the morning, when Forest Boy woke up, he reached out for them, and to his surprise, only one shoe was there. 'Where could his other shoe be?' he wondered. He put one shoe on and started hopping around, looking everywhere, all around his house in the hollow tree, and up and down the forest paths. But with no success!

I have lost a shoe, what am I to do! he cried.

Forest Boy then called on his friends, Baby Roo and Cockatoo, to come and help.

Baby Roo, Baby Roo, come and help me find my shoe!
Cockatoo, Cockatoo, come and help me find my shoe!

Baby Roo came bouncing and jumping along the path. Cockatoo came flying down from a high tree above.

When Baby Roo and Cockatoo heard what had happened, they both went off in search of the missing red shoe. Baby Roo bounced off the pathways and through the bushes. Cockatoo flew up and down and all around above Baby Roo's head.

After looking in many places, Baby Roo and Cockatoo, at exactly the same time, spied something *red* poking out of the bushes. Cockatoo flew down and Baby Roo jumped closer. They peered into the bushes, and there, fast asleep, in the middle of the red shoe, was a little brown mouse.

'Little mouse, what are you doing sleeping inside Forest Boy's red shoe?' cried Baby Roo and Cockatoo in one voice.

Little mouse woke up and looked out. 'Last night the rain fell down and washed away my house, so I looked and looked, and inside a hollow tree I found a new, very warm and very soft, red house!'

Baby Roo and Cockatoo laughed together. 'Little mouse, we need to help you make another house. This little red house is Forest Boy's shoe!'

So Baby Roo dug a new hole in the ground under some bushes, and Cockatoo gave some of his soft feathers to line the hole, and little brown mouse now had a new warm house to sleep in.

Then Baby Roo and Cockatoo took back the red shoe to give to Forest Boy. Forest Boy was so happy that he prepared some of his favourite fruits and nuts (and some sweet grasses for Baby Roo) and together they had a party to celebrate the finding of his lost red shoe.

Little brown mouse was also invited to the party, and from this day on (when he wasn't too busy sleeping inside his new warm house) he became a new friend of Forest Boy.

The Farmer and the Magic Stick

A traditional Masaii story narrated by Nenduvoto Nellie Mollel from Tanzania (transcribed by Susan Perrow). It concentrates on the rewards

of honesty rather than any punishments for dishonesty, and would be
suitable for telling to six- to ten-year-olds.

Once upon a time there was a man whose name was Eudin'malei. He
lived with his family on a small farm. One day, while he was walking
to the market to sell his produce, he met three men. They greeted each
other and Eudin'malei asked them 'Are you going to my house?' The
men replied 'No, no, no' and Eudin'malei replied, 'That is good, as I
hardly have enough rice to feed my family.' Then he started to sing:

> *Eudin'malei ai naata doye, naata doye, naata doye, tiatwe matata*
> *meiteu airono peji ndavadas tininam.* (Although I am poor I will
> be rich someday.)

Meanwhile the three men went straight to his house and ate all the
rice in the pot.
Eudin'malei continued with his journey to the market, and on
the way he met a lion. They greeted each other, and Eudin'malei
asked the lion 'Are you going to my house?' The lion replied 'No, no,
no' and Eudin'malei replied 'That is good, as my cow hardly gives
enough milk to feed my family.' Then he started to sing:

> *Eudin'malei ai naata doye, naata doye, naata doye, tiatwe matata*
> *meiteu airono peji ndavadas tininam.* (Although I am poor I will
> be rich someday.)

Meanwhile the lion went straight to the house and ate the milking cow.
Eudin'malei continued with his journey to the market, and on the
way he met a snake. They greeted each other, and Eudin'malei asked
the snake, 'Are you going to my house?' The snake replied 'No, no,
no' and Eudin'malei replied, 'That is good, as my chickens hardly
give enough eggs to feed my family.' Then he started to sing:

> *Eudin'malei ai naata doye, naata doye, naata doye, tiatwe matata*
> *meiteu airono peji ndavadas tininam.* (Although I am poor I will
> be rich someday.)

Meanwhile the snake went straight to his house and ate all the
chickens.
Eudin'malei finally reached the market and sold his produce and
set off back home. On his way he saw a shining stick next to the

road. He crossed over to pick it up, and then he asked the stick 'Who are you?' The stick answered, 'I am *Kiman enjani nelau engine negwany.*' (Around the bush with everything more.)

Eudin'malei was surprised and responded 'What a strange name!'

The stick continued: 'I am a magic stick – hold on to me and I can help improve your life!'

Eudin'malei continued home carrying the magic stick. As he walked he sang his song:

> *Eudin'malei ai naata doye, naata doye, naata doye, tiatwe matata meiteu airono peji ndavadas tininam.* (Although I am poor I will be rich someday.)

When he arrived at his farm, he was surprised to see that his house was changed into a big house, full of many sacks of rice. On his farm there was a barn full of many cows, goats and sheep. In his chicken house there were many chicks. Now he was very rich. He kept his magic stick on a special shelf in his new house, and everyday he sang to it:

> *Eudin'malei ai naata doye, naata doye, naata doye, tiatwe matata meiteu airono peji ndavadas tininam.* (Although I am poor I will be rich someday)

Eudin'malei lived happily on his farm with his family and his magic stick for the rest of his days.

The Peddler and his Caps

A story rewritten by Susan Perrow (author unknown) – a playful tale about a group of thieving monkeys who were dealt with by a simple but honest trick. Sometimes it is helpful for children to learn about 'honest' tricks. Suitable for four years and up, and very effective told with props (many caps on the storyteller's head!).

Once upon a time, who knows when and where, there was a peddler who travelled from town to town selling caps.

> *Caps for sale, caps for sale,*
> *green and red and yellow too,*
> *orange and all shades of blue.*

On top of his head the peddler wore his favourite old, brown cap. On top of the brown cap he put his green caps. On top of the green caps he put his red caps. On top of the red caps he put his yellow caps. On top of the yellow caps he put his orange caps. And on top of the orange caps he put the rest of his caps – in all shades of blue.

This was how the peddler carried his caps from town to town. When he reached a new town he would walk up and down the streets calling out,

Caps for sale, caps for sale,
green and red and yellow too,
orange and all shades of blue.

One afternoon the peddler arrived at a large shady tree at the edge of town. The sun was shining down so brightly that he decided to have a rest in the shade. He lifted all the caps down and balanced them up against the tree trunk (except for his old brown cap that always stayed on his head, even when he slept!). Then he lay down next to the tree and fell fast asleep.

He slept for a long time. When he woke up the first thing he did was to look for his caps. But they were no longer against the tree.

He looked to the left of him.

No caps.

He looked to the right of him.

No caps.

He looked behind the tree.

No caps.

Then he looked up into the tree and saw the tree was full of monkeys. There were monkeys sitting on every branch and every monkey had one of his caps on their heads.

'You cheeky monkeys,' he shouted, shaking his finger at them, 'you give me back my caps.' But the monkeys only shook their fingers back at him and shouted, 'Ttchch, ttchch, ttchch.'

'You cheeky monkeys,' he shouted, shaking the finger of his other hand at them, 'you give me back my caps.' But the monkeys only shook their fingers back at him and shouted, 'Ttchch, ttchch, ttchch.'

'You cheeky monkeys,' he shouted, stamping his right foot, 'you give me back my caps.' But the monkeys stood up on the branches and stamped their feet and shouted, 'Ttchch, ttchch, ttchch.'

'You cheeky monkeys,' he shouted, stamping his left foot, 'you give me back my caps.' But the monkeys stamped their other foot and shouted, 'Ttchch, ttchch, ttchch.'

The peddler was so angry that he took off his old brown cap and threw it on the ground.

Every monkey then took their cap off and threw it on the ground.

Now the peddler was able to gather up all his caps and stack them up on his head. On top of the brown cap he put his green caps. On top of the green caps he put his red caps. On top of the red caps he put his yellow caps. On top of the yellow caps he put his orange caps. And on top of the orange caps he put the rest of his caps – in all shades of blue.

Then the peddler walked back into the town, up and down the streets, calling out,

> *Caps for sale, caps for sale,*
> *green and red and yellow too,*
> *orange and all shades of blue.*

'Story bones' – The Silver Branch

At an Early Childhood Conference in Brisbane, a teacher presented the following 'story bones' for a story for a six-and-a-half-year-old girl who was always lying to cover up what she had done.

The story is about a monkey family that lived in the jungle – this family had a special branch at the top of a very high tree that had 'caught' so much moonlight over so many years that it had turned silver. It was a favourite place for anyone in the family to sit as it had special healing powers (examples of these powers could be listed here). One night one of the monkeys decided she wanted this branch just for herself – so she swung on it very hard till it broke off – then she took it away to hide it in a dense bush down below in the jungle. However, as soon as she reached the hiding place, the monkey saw that the silver light had gone from the branch – it just looked like an ordinary branch. What was she to do? She tried to take it back up to the top of the tree but couldn't find a way to make it stay there by itself … eventually a helper (Mother Moon?) gets involved and … (complete as you wish).

10

Divorce/Separation/Blended Families

A Family of Snails
by Matthew Barton

Note from the author: My grandson was born when my daughter was quite young, and they both lived with us for the first four years of his life. We were therefore very involved in caring for him. At a certain point, quite rightly, our daughter needed to establish her independence and move away. However this wasn't an easy transition for any of us. Our grandson was very attached to his 'old home' and we grandparents also found it a considerable wrench. Probably both his feelings and ours reinforced each other and accentuated the problem. I wrote this story to ease the transition and establish a sense of positive parting and, at the same time, continued connection. It is hard to say what effect the story had on our grandson, but he listened intently to it on several occasions and I was left with a feeling that it had 'gone in'. Strangely, writing the story also helped me in some way to acknowledge and come to terms with his departure. A strong connection has been maintained, and our grandson regularly and happily makes the short journey back and forth between his new home and his old.

Once upon a time there were five snails – 1, 2, 3, 4, 5 – living inside a snug flowerpot that the gardener had left in a shady corner of the garden. There was a grandma and a granddad snail, a mummy snail and a sweet little snail, and an uncle snail. The old flowerpot was quite big and there was room for all of them. It was cool, moist and beautifully slimy, and the grandma and mummy snails had made beautiful silvery pictures on the walls.

Every night, when the moon shone bright, the little snail went for a little slow slippery slide down to the gardener's lettuce bed, and had a nibble of this and a nibble of that. It was a lovely life, and the little snail was happy living in the snug flowerpot in the moist, shady corner of the big garden.

But one day his mummy came back from a long journey to the bottom of the garden. This was so far away the little snail had never even been there. Mummy snail was very excited. She said: 'I went down the path and over a tree stump and across a flowerbed and under a fern leaf and then – do you know what I found?' 'No,' said everyone, 'what did you find?' 'A big brick wall,' she said. 'Is that all,' they said. 'No it isn't,' she said. 'I slid up it and there I found a snuggly hole going right inside the wall, with little cracks for windows to see out of, and lovely soft moss to sleep on, and lots of different nooks and crannies. It's shady and moist and soft and nice. I'm going to go and live there with little snail.

So mummy snail and little snail and grandma snail and granddad snail, and uncle snail as well, all set off to see. They went down the path and over a tree stump and across a flowerbed and under a fern leaf, and then they came to the wall. They slid up it, and poked their delicate feelers into the cosy hole. Yes, it was very nice. Mummy snail was already making lovely silvery pictures everywhere, and little snail found a cosy chamber to sleep in. When he woke up the moon was shining bright, and granddad and grandma and uncle snail had gone back to their old flowerpot.

Sometimes little snail was a little bit sad that they didn't all live together any more – but whenever he wanted he could slip down the wall, go under the fern leaf, across the flower bed, over the tree stump and up the path to see his old flowerpot home. There it was! Still the same! Sometimes he went there; and sometimes grandma, granddad and uncle snail came to see him in his new hole-in-the-wall home. So he had two homes now. That was good. A nice moist flowerpot home and a cosy mossy wall home!

A home in a wall
And a home in a pot
And between them a silvery trail.
A home in a pot
And a home in a wall
Is really quite nice for a snail!

Big Things When You are Little
(A short story in two parts) by Natasha Hund

I have included the following as an example of how simple a 'healing' story can be. As Natasha has discovered, sharing family memory stories can be such a great way to ease anxiety in separated family situations.

Note from Natasha: I am responding to a post on your FaceBook page asking for stories people have written after experiencing your work. I did your Storytelling unit at SCU as part of my Grad Dip., specializing in Play. As part of that I wrote the attached family story for my daughter. Her father and I are separated and through the story I wanted to connect her to some of our childhood memories, and bring a sense of unity. With her father not present in the household I used stories to keep his presence alive outside the times she spent with him. Also I come from a family of Dutch immigrants and did not have extended family here in Australia, and as a child I loved to hear stories of my parents' homeland and families. I also wanted to share this with my daughter as she grew up so she would have a sense and knowledge of her ancestry.

Mummy's story: When I was little, my mum (your Oma) used to take me for a walk every day. On our walks we would visit the playground and parks, but I especially loved to visit the animals. Near where we lived there was a paddock where I could watch the goats and horses eat grass. I know all the animals that lived near our house: Boffie our cat, Poukie our dog, the turtle the children had a couple of houses down, and all of the wonderful insects and birds in our garden.

One day as we were going on our walk, I saw a man taking a horse for a walk on a leash. 'Horse,' I proudly informed Oma. Oma saw what I was looking at and replied, 'No Natasha, it's a doggie.' It was in fact a huge Great Dane. 'Horse,' I repeated. Oma tried to correct me again, 'No Natasha, it's a doggie.' Well, I got that determined look on my face like you sometimes have, and with great authority declared again, 'Horse.'

Oma realized there was no use in arguing with me, so that day the Great Dane indeed became a horse!

Daddy's story: When daddy was a little boy, about four years old, he went on a really long plane trip to the other side of the world. He went to the country where his mother and father were born. With daddy's mother, your Nona, daddy stayed in the village where Nona was born, and her own mother before that. The village had beautiful stone buildings that had been there for centuries, there was a creek with clear fresh water, and green rolling hills surrounded the village on all sides.

Daddy made friends with one of the dogs at the village and they would play together. One day, being adventurous as he is, daddy went for a walk into the cornfields. He enjoyed exploring the fields; looking at the tall stalks and their cobs of corn, and the dirt and insects. He also had the dog for company. When daddy tried to get out of the cornfields he realized he did not know where he was and could not see the village because the corn was so tall. Even when you are a grown-up the corn is taller than your head so you can imagine how tall it would seem to a four-year-old boy. Daddy called out to Nona, but no one seemed to hear him. It was frightening not to know how to get home, especially in a strange country. As it was starting to get dark, daddy's dog friend finally led him home, maybe the dog was getting hungry for dinner. Daddy must have felt relieved to be amongst familiar surroundings and people. He told me he never went into the cornfields again after that. When Daddy told me his story he said, 'The cornfields were too big.'

Saturdays

A childhood memory story

Sometimes in family life, when siblings are fighting and things are chaotic, a memory story of the good times when the parents were children can be just what is needed. It can help soothe the situation and be a gentle reminder that families have special times as well as difficult times. This is one example of such a memory story – from my own childhood.

I was born in Tamworth, a country town in Australia, and I spent the first ten years of my life growing up in a house at the foot of the hills behind the town.

Saturdays were my best memory.

Not the first part of Saturday, as this is when the jobs had to be done! Many jobs! My older brother David had outside things to do – trimming the hedges, weeding the garden, that sort of thing. I had inside things to do – washing up, mopping the floor, dusting, that sort of thing. David used to call me 'Rapunzel' as I was always inside the 'castle' doing things while he was always outside.

But late morning, when the jobs were finished, our mother would give us a rucksack and we would head off into the hills behind the house. Inside the rucksack were two packages – some sausages wrapped in paper, and some buttered bread wrapped in paper. There was also a bottle of water and two coloured metal cups, and a box of matches. Sometimes, on a lucky day, as well as water we had a bottle of lemonade or fizzy orange.

It was adventure time! It was the time we both looked forward to all week.

I think I must have been about eight when these adventures started, and my brother was three years older than me. So he was the one who carried the rucksack and he was the one in charge! We would make our way up the rocky gullies, David leading the way. We had a purpose – to find a good place to build a fire to cook our lunch. A good place meant one with large flat rocks and no grass close by or overhanging trees that could catch alight.

Once our fireplace had been found we set to work gathering dry sticks and branches, and choosing forked green sticks for cooking the sausages. Some of the wrapping paper was used to get the fire going, and some was kept to help protect our precious bread from invading ants. Once the fire had settled down a little, we squatted around it with our sausage precariously balanced on the forked stick, trying to cook it evenly on every side. Of course, this was an impossible task. Invariably we ended up eating half-cooked meat; or, if the sausage had fallen into the fire, some very burnt meat, if not pure charcoal. But for some strange reason, once the sausage (raw or burnt or both) was wrapped in the buttered bread, it always tasted wonderful.

On one occasion, one of David's sausages burst open and the 'guts' (middle) spilled out into the fire. For weeks after this event, we would dissolve into laughter at the dinner table when my brother whispered to me, 'Remember the day when the guts fell out of the sausage?' Our parents never understood how we could laugh so much about nothing!

Once lunch was over, we used a mixture of water and dirt to put out the fire, and then packed up our rucksack. With our tummies full, we now had the rest of the afternoon to play. There seemed to be an endless line of hills and gullies to explore, and we were always on the lookout for pepper trees to climb, caves to hide in and pools of water amongst the dry hot rocks.

It was rare that the gullies had any water. Usually the creek beds were dry, but occasionally we would come across a shallow pool that glistened like a shining mirror. We would pretend we had reached the ocean and dip our hands into it to enjoy the coolness of the water. Tamworth was a long way from the coast and we often fantasized about living by the sea (it is interesting that we both ended up raising our own families within walking distance of the ocean).

Late in the afternoon we would arrive home – tired, dirty, and sometimes with scratched and burnt fingers. But, always so happy to have had such an adventure!

In another week, Saturday would come round again. After doing our jobs, up into the gullies we would go, with the rucksack on David's back and our 'lunch' wrapped up in paper parcels inside.

Yes, this was definitely one of my best childhood memories.

The Children and the Butterfly

A Tanzanian story told by Salma Haji Mnubi at a teacher-training module in Nairobi and transcribed by Susan Perrow. This African fairytale has a similar theme to Hansel *and* Gretel, *with wonderful images of a brother and sister separated from their home and parents, working together to find their way out of danger and safely back home. Suitable for 5–8 year olds.*

> *Twende tukawinde leo, Twende tukawinde leo,*
> *Tukaa winde vipepeo, Tukaa winde vipepeo,*
> *Ai mama vipepeo, vipepeo.*

(Let's go hunting today, let's go hunting today; hunting for butterflies; Ai mama, butterflies, butterflies.)

Once upon a time there were two children, a boy and a girl, and they lived with their parents near the forest. The boy was called Dudu and the girl was called Raya.

One day as they were playing outside their house, a beautiful butterfly came fluttering around the flowers. It fluttered all around and then flew up and out of the garden. Raya and her brother Dudu saw it and stopped what they had been doing. Then together they started to follow the butterfly, singing:

> *Twende tukawinde leo, Twende tukawinde leo,*
> *Tukaa winde vipepeo, Tukaa winde vipepeo,*
> *Ai mama vipepeo, vipepeo.*

The butterfly flew up and past the neighbour's house; and Dudu and Raya followed it. The butterfly flew further and further away from their house, deep into the forest, but Dudu and Raya were still behind it, following. After a while both of them grew tired of running after the butterfly and they wanted to go back. But because they had been running without knowing where they were going, they realized that they were now lost, and neither of them knew the way home.

Then, in a clearing, they saw a house, a very small house, with walls made of biscuits, and roof made of bread. They went and knocked on the door, but no one answered. Dudu tried the door and it opened. They went in, but nobody was home. Because they were very hungry they decided to eat the wall of the house that was made of biscuits. They ate until their stomachs were full.

As they were resting after their meal, the owner of the house returned home. It was an old woman who was very angry when she saw that her walls had been eaten by Raya and Dudu, so she told them that she was going to eat one of them. She chose Dudu to be her prize – after he had grown fat.

The old woman put Dudu in a room with a door which had a little hole in it. She told Dudu that every day he had to show his hand through the hole so she would know whether he was growing fat. The old woman locked the door and off she went outside.

Time passed and Dudu, fed on biscuits and bread, grew fatter and fatter. Meanwhile Raya was kept busy doing jobs for the old woman, but always she kept an eye out for a way to help free her brother. One day her chance came when the old woman dropped the key to Dudu's room without knowing.

Raya saw the key and put it in her pocket. When the old woman was sleeping she quickly opened the door for her brother and off they ran, away from the house. At first they seemed lost in the forest again, but then they saw the butterfly, the same butterfly they had followed before. They ran after it as it flew in and out of the trees. They ran and ran, until the butterfly led them out of the forest and back home.

Their parents, who had been crying because of their lost children, welcomed them back with open arms. Raya and Dudu told their parents the whole story and promised them that they would never wander far from home again. Their mother and father were very happy to have their children back safe and sound, and they lived happily together from that day onwards.

Twende tukawinde leo, Twende tukawinde leo,
Tukaa winde vipepeo, Tukaa winde vipepeo,
Ai mama vipepeo, vipepeo.

Little Brown Bulb

A 'warming' story for three- to five-year-olds about finding HOME! This story could be used as a basis for many versions of a little one looking for 'home' – e.g. replacing the bulb with something else that is looking for a home (say a puppy; or baby turtle that needs to find its way to the sea; or a baby bird that has fallen from the tree and needs to find its nest again … etc.). In the repeated rhyme, if appropriate, 'mother' can also be replaced by 'father'.

A little brown bulb was lost in the autumn garden. She wandered from plant to plant, from flower to flower, crying out:

> *Where is my mother, where is my home,*
> *Where is a bed I can call my own?*

She looked up and around and around about.
She saw a spider weaving his web of silver bright. She asked the spider:

> *Can you help me find my mother, can you help me find my home,*
> *Can you help me find a bed I can call my own?*

But the spider shook his head – 'I'm too busy trying to catch my autumn dinner to help *you*, little brown bulb.'
So the little brown bulb wandered on. She looked up and around and around about. She saw a lizard lying on top of a large brown rock. She asked the lizard:

> *Can you help me find my mother, can you help me find my home,*
> *Can you help me find a bed I can call my own?*

But the lizard shook his head – 'I'm too busy trying to soak up the last rays of the summer sun to help *you*, little brown bulb.'
So the little brown bulb wandered on. She looked up and around and around about. She saw a willy-wagtail poking her head out of a hole in the fence post. She asked the willy-wagtail:

> *Can you help me find my mother, can you help me find my home,*
> *Can you help me find a bed I can call my own?*

But the willy-wagtail shook her head – 'I'm too busy trying to build my nest for winter to help *you*, little brown bulb.'

So the little brown bulb wandered on until she came to a golden cassia tree. She sat down amongst the golden petals under the tree and began to cry.

Then she heard a creeping, shuffling sound and a little voice said to her: 'Whatever is the matter little brown bulb? Perhaps I can help?'

Little brown bulb wiped her eyes and saw Hairy Caterpillar in front of her. 'I'm lost!' she said, 'I can't find my mother, I can't find my home, I can't find a bed I can call my own!'

'Well, well,' said Hairy Caterpillar, 'You haven't been looking in the right place. You have been looking up and around and around about, but if you looked DOWN you would see that your mother is waiting with open arms for you. Now follow me!'

Then Hairy Caterpillar wriggled under some golden flower petals and down into the ground between two rocks. The little brown bulb followed, and soon, so soon, she found herself in the arms of Mother Earth, right where she belonged. Mother Earth then closed her arms, covering the little brown bulb with a warm blanket of rich brown soil. And the little brown bulb, who was so tired from all her wanderings, closed her eyes and fell fast asleep, snug in her new earth home.

She slept for a very, very, very long time – all through the cold winter months – and she didn't wake up until the springtime – but that is another story: a flower story!

The Magic Cooking Pot

A Xhosa story from South Africa transcribed by Esther Mini and Susan Perrow. It is a wonderful tale to help reassure children about how special they are, and can offer affirming, soothing story medicine in a world of turmoil and change, especially family changes. Suitable for ages 4–8.

Once upon a time, in a village in a faraway land, a woman called Nozuko lived by herself. Her home was a rondavel – a round mud brick hut with a thatched roof and brightly painted walls. Her work each day was in the fields – digging the ground, planting maize, pulling up weeds – and she grew the biggest, best-tasting maize in the whole village, and she baked the best-tasting corn bread in the whole village! She was a good, hardworking woman, and she was happy with her life – except for one thing! She had always wanted her house to be filled with the laughter of little children, and yet all her life she had lived alone and her house was silent.

One day Nozuko decided to go and visit the 'sangoma', the magic man, and tell him her problem. His house was a long walk from the village, on the other side of the river, so Nozuko set off early, before the hot sun had climbed too high in the sky. She wrapped up her best loaf of golden corn bread to take with her. Following the path down to the river, she crossed the stepping stones (stopping for a cool drink on her way), then continued on the long path up the hill to the sangoma's house. As she walked she sang:

Sifikil' ezibukweni, dancu, dancu siwelile, masisele emanzini.
(I arrive at the river, I jump across the stones, then I drink some water)

When she reached the sangoma's house, the sangoma was sitting outside waiting for her. He was wearing his magic hat, made of many coloured feathers, and he had a large leather pouch tied at his waist. When Nozuko told him of her wish for her house to be filled with the laughter of little children, he tipped the stones out of his pouch and they rolled into a pattern on the ground in front of him.

For a long time Nozuko waited while the sangoma sat looking at the pattern of stones, then finally he looked up at her and said, 'Yes, I can help you but you must do as I say. Firstly, go back to your house and fill your big black cooking pot with water, then light a fire under it to boil the water. While the water is boiling, go out and gather as many different fruits as you can find and bring them back and put them in your cooking pot. Then you must wait outside your house while the fruits are cooking in the pot, and when you can smell they are ready, go inside and you will see what you will see.'

Nozuko thanked the sangoma by giving him the golden corn bread, then she set off back home, down the windy hill-side path to the river, across the stepping stones (stopping for a cool drink on the way), and all the way back to her village. And as she walked she sang:
Sifikil' ezibukweni, dancu, dancu siwelile, masisele emanzini.
When she reached her house she started to do exactly what the sangoma had told her. Firstly she filled her big black cooking pot with water, then stacked wood under it and lit the fire. Then she put a large basket on her head and walked to the village orchard. There she picked a pawpaw, a banana, a mango, an orange, a narchie (mandarin), a pineapple and a granadilla (passion fruit), and carefully placed them in the basket. When she arrived back at her house, the water was already boiling, so she added the fruit to the water, put some more wood on the fire, and then went outside to sit and wait in the shade of the African flame tree that grew by her front door.

Well children, Nozuko must have been so tired from all her hard work, that while she was waiting she fell asleep … and she slept a very long time! When she woke up, the first thing she noticed was the beautiful smell coming from inside her house. She quickly jumped up and opened the door, and there, to her great surprise, she saw two children sitting in front of the fire.

Nozuko sat down and hugged each child, and then she was so happy she started to laugh … and the children climbed into her lap and started to laugh as well …

Now if you ever visit Nozuko's village you will know which house is hers because you can always hear the happy laughter of children, and you can often hear this song:

> *Sifikil' ezibukweni, dancu, dancu siwelile, masisele emanzini.*

'Story bones' – penguins, towers, toadstools and canoes

There are so many different situations with separated families and each story requires 'tailoring' if it is to have any chance of helping the situation. Here are the bones from four such situations, for you to work with and expand into stories, or to give you ideas for your own story-making.

The Penguin Family

A story for a six-year-old living in two different households with two different sets of rules, but loved and safe in both.

A large family of penguins lived on an iceberg that floated round the deep blue ocean at the top of the world. For a long time life continued with very few interruptions – the penguins ate, they slept, they played, and the next day they ate, they slept and they played some more. But one day there was a great storm and huge waves lashed at the edges of the iceberg. The iceberg bobbed up and down with the waves, and then, all of a sudden, the strength of the waves caused a large crack to appear right across the middle of the ice and the iceberg split in half …

The Two Towers

A story for an eight-year-old boy with separated parents to encourage the child to go to visit the other parent.

Story about a kingdom with two towers and one prince – great storm and earthquake splits the two towers, creating a large ravine – the wind from the storm blows all memories into the ravine – then armies escort the prince across a bridge over the ravine – now it is an exciting adventure to visit the other tower and return back again – (and how does he recover the memories?)

The Storm and the Toadstool

A story for a five-year-old child who is anxious about visiting the father who lives quite far away

A story about a magic toadstool and the fairy family that lived under it – storm breaks toadstool in half and lifts one half up and puts it down in another part of the forest. Child fairy wants to visit father in other part of forest – wind fairy helps guide the way.

A Canoe Story

A story for two stepbrothers who always quarrel and cannot get on

A story about a family that is going on a long journey down a river – each family member has their own canoe (with their own bed) – all the canoes are tied together when the river is wide and flowing easily – if one canoe tips (or is pushed over) it affects all the others. But sometimes the river passage is quite thin and full of rapids so each canoe has to be untied and 'go it alone'.

A helping metaphor could be the 'magic' paddle that each family member has carved for themselves before leaving on their journey – perhaps each one has carved a special design, an animal totem, some symbols and wishes to guide and guard them on their way.

The paddle belonging to each person helps in many different ways on the journey – going down the rapids, when stuck in the reeds and bushes close to the bank, to ward off crocodiles and other dangerous animals on the way, to keep balance, to link the canoes together, etc.

A wonderful strengthening experience for this storyline would be for the family with the stepchildren to go on a real canoe journey, and all carve designs in their paddles before setting out.

11

Fussiness/Complaining

Winnie the Fussy Eater
by Shan Ang

Shan's comments after telling her three-year-old son the story: 'Now he eats the vegetables but still does not eat fruits except apple and banana so I think the story worked ... but at least he is able to accept green vegetables better.' My response was 'The story was about a rainbow vegetable garden, not a fruit orchard, so it did its healing work beautifully!'

Winnie the Pooh ate nothing each day except honey. Then it happened that it rained for days. It rained and rained and rained and the bees were short of honey. As a result, Winnie got hungrier and hungrier until his eyes began to see stars and his legs felt like jelly. His friends tried to offer him some fruits, nuts and vegetables. But Winnie always said 'no' because he only wanted honey.

Winnie's friends were worried about how weak he had become, and they decided to ask the old owl for help. The owl told Winnie and his friends there was a magical garden in the forest that could help him become strong again. With the help of his friends, Winnie made his way to the magical garden.

When they were in the forest, they heard a beautiful chorus coming from nearby.

> *There is a secret nobody knows, something in us that helps you grow. Try us morning, noon and night, and we will make you strong and bright.*

There, in front of them, was a rainbow-coloured garden filled with orange carrots, green lettuce, red tomatoes, yellow sweetcorn and purple eggplants, cheerfully singing.

A rabbit came hopping along and sang:

Juicy juicy lettuce – Can I have some so that I can have strong legs
when I hop?

'Yes you may,' cried the lettuce.
So the rabbit took some and hopped happily away.
A monkey came to sit on a tree and sang:

Juicy juicy tomato – can I have some so that I can have quick limbs
when I climb?

'Yes you may' cried the tomatoes.
So the monkey took some and climbed happily away.
A chick came along and sang:

Juicy juicy sweetcorn – can I have some so that I can be strong and
steady as daddy rooster?

'Yes you may,' cried the corn
So the chick took some and ran happily away.
Winnie the Pooh could not wait any more. He wanted to hop,
climb and be strong and steady.
So he came forward and sang:

Juicy juicy lettuce,
Juicy juicy tomato,
Juicy juicy sweetcorn, can I have some so that
my legs can be strong like the rabbit,
my limbs can be quick like the monkey,
my mind strong and steady like the rooster?

'Yes you may,' cried the lettuce, tomato and sweetcorn, in unison.
Winnie the Pooh took some of each vegetable and with every bite
he felt strength returning to his weak hands and legs. Soon he was
able to walk home without help from his friends.
From this time onwards, Winnie remembered to eat something
from the magic garden every day; and sometimes he still has a little
honey for dessert!

The White Birds and the Rain

This is a story about the wonder of rain and water – written to encourage children to drink water instead of asking for sweetened drinks every time they are thirsty. The story was inspired by an intricately carved Chinese scene set in a glass box, with mountains and valleys and two white cranes feeding in the grasses by a curved wooden bridge. I had bought the carving for my grandson's sixth birthday, and the story was written as an encouragement for him to drink more water (a wish of his parents).

There was once a young boy who loved the rain. He loved to dance in the silver raindrops, he loved to jump in the muddy rain puddles, and he loved to drink the fresh rainwater as it fell from the sky.

This boy lived in a land where every afternoon the rain clouds would appear high in the sky and soon the raindrops would fall down from the clouds and into his garden. Every day he was able to dance in the silver raindrops, jump in the muddy rain puddles, and drink the fresh rainwater as it fell from the sky.

But one day, even though the rain clouds filled the sky, the raindrops didn't fall. The boy waited until the next day, and the next day, and the next day, and still no rain fell from the clouds high up in the sky.

'If I could only fly', the boy thought, 'I would fly up to the clouds and find a way to shake out the rain, so the raindrops can fall on my garden again.'

But the boy did not have wings, so he could not fly. He decided to ask one of his flying friends to help. He went out into his garden to see what flying friends were there.

First he saw a Lady Beetle:

Lady Beetle, Lady Beetle, fly up high;
Fly to the clouds at the top of the sky.
Find a way to shake out the rain,
So the raindrops can fall on my garden again.

But Lady Beetle answered:

My wings are too small to fly so high; I can't fly up to the top of the sky.
Why don't you ask the butterfly, her wings can help her fly up high.

So the boy called out to Butterfly:

Butterfly, Butterfly, fly up high;
Fly to the clouds at the top of the sky.
Find a way to shake out the rain,
So the raindrops can fall on my garden again.

But Butterfly answered:

My wings are too small to fly so high; I can't fly up to the top of the sky.
Why don't you ask the Black Crow, her wings can help her fly up high.

So the boy called out to Black Crow:

Black Crow, Black Crow, fly up high;
Fly to the clouds at the top of the sky.
Find a way to shake out the rain,
So the raindrops can fall on my garden again.

But Black Crow answered:

My wings are too small to fly so high; I can't fly up to the top of the sky.
Why don't you ask the giant white cranes, their giant wings can help
them fly up high, all the way to the top of the sky.

Now the boy had never heard of the giant white cranes, so he asked Black Crow where he could find them.

'Down in the valley, below your garden, there is a path that curves over a bridge. Below the bridge you will find the home of the white cranes,' said Black Crow.

So the boy set out walking, out from his garden and down through the valley, until he reached a path that curved over a bridge. When he looked down below the bridge, standing in the reeds were two beautiful white birds, larger than any birds he had ever seen before.

'Excuse me,' said the boy, 'are you the giant white cranes with giant wings that can fly so high?'

The cranes replied together, 'Yes, our wings are so wide we can fly all the way to the top of the sky!'

The boy then told them that the clouds had stopped raining and he was searching for a way to bring back the raindrops. Perhaps they could help?

White cranes, white cranes, fly up high;
Fly to the clouds at the top of the sky.
Find a way to shake out the rain,
So the raindrops can fall on my garden again.

The white cranes were very happy to help. They spread their wide wings and set out, flying high, so high, all the way to where the clouds were floating, heavy with rain, at the top of the sky. When the cranes reached the clouds, they tickled and shook them with their long feathers, and poked holes in them with their long beaks. After much tickling and poking, the clouds could no longer hold all their water in, and they started to let the raindrops fall down.

Down in the world below, the boy had just returned to his garden. Suddenly he felt pitter-patter, splish-splash, drip-drop! The rain was falling again! He was so happy. Once again he could dance in the silver raindrops, jump in the muddy rain puddles, and drink the fresh rainwater as it fell from the sky.

'Thank-you white cranes', he called out to the giant birds as they flew back across the sky.

From that day on, whenever the clouds held back the rain, the boy knew that all he had to do was visit his new flying friends down in the valley below and ask them to help. The white cranes would then spread their wings and fly high, so high, all the way to where the clouds were floating, heavy with rain, at the top of the sky.

When the white cranes reached the clouds, they would tickle and shake them with their long feathers, and poke holes in them with their long beaks. After much tickling and poking, the clouds could no longer hold all their water in. They would let their raindrops fall down, down, down, all the way down to the world below, down to where the children would dance in the silver raindrops, jump in the muddy rain puddles, and drink the fresh rainwater as it fell from the sky.

Little Wolf
by Kim Davie

Note from the author: I worked on this story – for a complaining, uncooperative child – whilst Susan was lecturing our class as part of our teacher-training/therapeutic storytelling module. The child in question was unwilling to participate in social and learning situations, continually complaining that things were not to his liking. It was written for the middle childhood age range 9 to 12 (as reflected in the 'rap' language used by Little Wolf). I have some knowledge of wolves and their pack behaviour, so I decided to use 'Little Wolf' as my main character.

Little Wolf sat outside the den whining and yipping. Shards of light speared through the trees and pierced the forest floor as the morning sun climbed over the distant, eastern mountains.

'What's the matter Little Wolf?' His mother trotted up to him, dropping a freshly killed rabbit at his feet and licking his face. 'What brings you out of the cosy den so early in the morning?'

'Ergh, Mum, don't do that, it's wet!'

Mother Wolf laughed, 'But Little Wolf, that's how we wolves always greet each other, it's our clan's tradition. You must now acknowledge my lick with a nudge, muzzle to muzzle, as a sign of your love and respect.'

'It's a stupid sign and I won't do it. I'm out here in the cold because my brothers are snoring and there are too many of us for that small den. I want my own den, I'm big enough now. I don't like sharing it with all those other cubs, and, you've brought rabbit home again. I'm sick of rabbit.'

'Little Wolf, you must learn the language and signs of our clan. You must learn of the dangers that lie in the great forest before the time of midwinter moon and the first cub hunt. Only after you have proved yourself a useful pack member and helped bring down prey can you dig your own den and seek a mate in the camp.'

But Little Wolf put his paws over his ears, closed his eyes and began a whining chant.

> *I'm Little Wolf, bored as can be.*
> *Everyone is having fun, everyone but me.*
> *My den is cramped, it's way too small,*
> *I don't know why I stay at all.*
> *The food is dull, the clan is dumb,*
> *My life is dreary, Listen Mum!*

Mother Wolf sighed. She loved Little Wolf very much and wanted him to be happy like the other cubs in the pack. Every day they ran around the camp, pouncing and wrestling, learning the hunt signals, preparing themselves for the midwinter moon hunt when they would be allowed to join in for the first time with bringing down the prey. But Little Wolf didn't want to try. He never joined in when the other cubs played pouncing hide-and-seek games. Instead, he sat outside the den and yipped his whining chant.

> *I'm Little Wolf, bored as can be.*
> *Everyone is having fun, everyone but me.*
> *The light's too bright, my eyes can't see,*
> *Go and play your stupid games, but don't ask me.*
> *The sun's too hot, the pouncing's dumb,*
> *You can ask me all you like but I won't come!*

Pretty soon the other cubs tired of Little Wolf's complaints and stopped asking him to play. This made Mother Wolf sad. She worried that when the midwinter moon came, Little Wolf would not be ready to join in the hunt with the rest of the pack. So each day she spent time teaching him what she could to help him grow and learn the ways of the wolf clan. Little Wolf, however, seldom listened and would wander off whenever he could to whine and yip to whoever would listen.

> *I'm Little Wolf, as bored as can be*
> *Everyone is having fun, no one's asking me*
> *The grass is dry, the trees are brown*
> *Around the camp the leaves fall down*
> *The day's too short, the night's too long*
> *The sun's not warm, everything is wrong.*

The days were indeed growing shorter and the time of midwinter moon soon came. The cubs were excited. They had practised all summer and autumn and now they were ready for their first hunt.

'Stay close Little Wolf,' whispered Mother Wolf as the pack gathered together and began to move out from the camp, alert for the signs of prey. 'Listen, watch and sniff. Be ready for the leader's signal and move swiftly, for the hunt will take us far from camp.' But Little Wolf was too busy whining and yipping to listen to his mother's warning.

> *I'm Little Wolf, as bored as can be*
> *Everyone is having fun, everyone but me*
> *The trot's too fast, there is no prey*
> *Why can't we hunt on another day?*
> *The snow is cold, the air is damp*
> *I want to go right back to camp.*

Suddenly, there was a yip and a yap from the pack leader and all around him wolves began to run. 'Little Wolf, let's go!' his mother called.

But Little Wolf had sat down in the snow, his paws over his ears, eyes squeezed shut – as he always did when things were not to his liking (and they seldom were).

This hunt is hard, don't want to run.
Why can't I ever have some fun?

He waited for his mother's patient lick.

Nothing happened.

Little Wolf opened one eye. He couldn't see his mother, in fact, he couldn't see any wolves at all. He listened carefully, straining his ears but the soft footfalls of the pack had faded. He lifted his snout, sniffed the breeze and tasted the air. He thought he caught just the faintest whiff of wolf scent and then … it was gone.

Little Wolf shivered. For the first time in his life he was really alone. The wind blew stronger and the woods grew dark as the moon slipped behind a cloud. Suddenly, something rustled in the bushes right behind him.

Little Wolf didn't wait to find out what it was. He turned and ran as fast as he could back towards the camp. He kept on running until he was out of breath, but when he stopped and looked around him the camp was nowhere in sight. Everything looked and smelled strange. All was quiet. Then he smelled a familiar scent – fresh prey.

Little Wolf pressed his snout close to the ground and began to follow the scent – slowly at first, then more quickly as his hunger grew. He reached a clearing and there in the centre lay a large chunk of deer meat. Little Wolf trotted right up to the meat ready for a tasty treat. He was feeling pretty pleased with himself for having found this prey without any help. He took a step closer and opened his mouth but instead of the mouthwatering taste of sweet meat he felt a tug on his leg and a sharp twinge as a cord tightened around his paw.

Little Wolf yipped in surprise and alarm. He jumped and pulled and rolled around on the snowy ground but the cord held fast. He tried to bite the cord but his leg was pulled behind and he couldn't reach. However he tried he could not loosen the cord – he was stuck fast.

Little Wolf lay in the snow. He opened his mouth to yip and whine but then he stopped.

There was no one to hear. He put his head on his paws and sighed. He longed for his mother and his pack. He didn't like the strange smells and the quiet of this place. It felt wrong. What was he to do?

High in the branches of a nearby tree an owl hooted softly. Little Wolf felt a strange feeling welling up inside him, and then a sound began deep inside his belly, a soft rumbling that grew stronger and louder inside him until he felt as if he would burst right open. He sat up, threw his head back and opened his throat wide. What do you think? The most amazing, long, lonely howl echoed through the woods.

Little Wolf was so surprised that he just sat there. Then, in the distance, he heard a faint answering howl. Then another and another. He threw back his head and howled again, this time adding an excited yip at the end.

The answering howls grew louder and stronger and then stopped abruptly. Little Wolf waited, then he saw a set of shining yellow eyes on the edge of the clearing. The pack leader crept quietly around the clearing sniffing the breeze. Then he raised his head and yipped softly. Two more wolves joined him and one began to chew at the length of cord that held Little Wolf's leg. Before too long his sharp teeth had severed the rope. The knot loosened and fell apart, and Little Wolf was free.

The leader licked Little Wolf's face and nudged him gently towards the edge of the clearing. Then the wolves began to run. This time Little Wolf ran with them. He ran as fast as he could to stay close to the warm bodies of his pack. Far behind them in the distance his keen ears heard the snapping of twigs and the heavy footfall of boots as the hunter hurried to claim his wolf pelt.

In time the rescue party joined the rest of the pack and there were many joyful licks and yips for Little Wolf. This time Little Wolf didn't mind at all, he yipped and nudged happily with the rest of the pack. Mother Wolf was very proud of Little Wolf. 'What a clear and strong voice you have, Little Wolf. You will surely be a very useful member of the hunting party now.'

Little Wolf was very happy to be back safe in the camp with his pack. He didn't even complain when his brothers snored loudly in the den that night. He lay awake and thought of a new chant to sing when the sun came up. He couldn't wait to teach it to all his friends.

I'm Little Wolf as happy as can be.
Everyone is having fun, but no one more than me.
The sun is up, a brand new day,

So come on friends, let's yip and play.
We'll learn our wolf clan signs and soon,
We'll hunt with our pack in the light of the moon.

Then he snuggled up close to his brothers' warm, furry bodies and fell into a deep and peaceful sleep.

Little Elephant Does Not Want to Walk
by Erika Katacic Kozic

Note from the author: I am a chemist in Zagreb, Croatia, who enjoys storytelling and playing the didgeridoo. Occasionally I visit libraries, preschools and schools as a storyteller. 'Didgstories', my latest programme for children, includes storytelling with didgeridoo. The story 'Little Elephant Does Not Want to Walk' was written for story-telling with musical accompaniment using the guidelines for thera-peutic story formats. It is my first story written using help from your book, Healing Stories for Challenging Behaviour. *Inspiration for the story's theme came from my weekend hikes with my family and friends, during which a child sometimes lagged behind and whined, 'Are we there yet?' In this story, Little Elephant's friend thinks up a creative solution to make walking more fun. While travelling to the great lake, a herd of elephants and a flock of ox-pecker birds listen to him whine and whine. An ox-pecker solves the problem with a creative solution, weaving special nest-like slippers just for Little Elephant.*

After hearing the story, children could weave ribbons and bells into their laces and dance to the elephants' song. When out walking, ideas from the story could be used to encourage children to keep on going. For example, a walking game could be played where children march like elephants and sing along. While walking in the woods or park, they could search for interesting stems and twigs to make their own creations just like the ox-pecker did. Walking with rhythm and a song is always more fun than just plain walking.

For my first storytelling performance of 'Little Elephant Does Not Want to Walk', my colleague and I visited Daktil, a music preschool in Zagreb. To introduce the story, I asked the children if they ever had to walk a lot. All of them nodded yes. None of them, however, had any ideas about what to do when tired of walking. I then told the story while my colleague tooted along on the didgeridoo. The children immediately picked up on the rhythm, and some even swayed lightly and sang along. As soon as I had finished telling the story, one girl jumped up and exclaimed, 'I like the song!' We agreed she could sing it next time she went for a walk with her family. One boy said he would ask his mom to tell him this story while out walking together. Since my sons are almost in their teens, they are now too old for such simple stories. Nevertheless they did read it for a home quality-control test. After some laughter and giggling, they decided to try out the elephant march themselves on our next family hiking trip.

In the plains of Africa where the big animals graze, there is a bird known as the ox-pecker. Ox-peckers often perch on the backs of rhinoceros, antelope, zebras, and even elephants. They love eating the bugs that make these larger animals itch and scratch a lot. The grazing animals like ox-peckers because these birds keep them pest-free. Sometimes the big animals need to walk far in search of grass to eat and water to drink. The ox-peckers then travel with them, perched on their backs.

This is a story about a little elephant on a journey with his family and ox-peckers in Africa.

*

It was the dry season in Africa, and the elephants were on a journey to the great lake. They had already been walking for days, marching in a slow rhythm. To make their journey more fun, the big elephants thought up a marching song.

> *Elephants are we*
> *Marching happily*
> *We toot our song*
> *As we go along*
> *For elephants are we!*

But Little Elephant was not having any fun. Little Elephant did not like walking. He especially did not like going on journeys. So while the big elephants walked and sang, Little Elephant walked and whined.

Every so often Little Elephant would tug on his mommy's tail with his little trunk. Then he would cry, 'Are we there yet, mommy? I don't want to walk, mommy. My legs hurt, mommy. Can you carry me, mommy?'

Mommy Elephant would just reply, 'We have to walk, son. Because we need to reach the great lake where there is a lot of food to eat and water to drink. Sing with us, dear. It will make walking more fun.'

But Little Elephant did not feel like singing. So Little Elephant would walk and whine, walk and whine, while all the other elephants were walking and singing.

Elephants are we
Marching happily
We toot our song
As we go along
For elephants are we!

While Little Elephant walked and whined, his friend the ox-pecker listened to him and felt sorry for him. So he sang to Little Elephant and encouraged him to keep walking. But that was not enough. Little Elephant did not stop whining.

One day, the ox-pecker had a great idea and flew off during their noontime break. While Little Elephant rested in the shade, the ox-pecker gathered branches and wove new slippers just for Little Elephant. He wove in soft leaves and blades of grass, and shaped the slippers into four little nests. Then one by one, the ox-pecker carried the woven slippers to Little Elephant.

'Hey buddy, I have a present for you! You are little, and the journey is long. So I wove these slippers out of branches, leaves, and grass, to make walking more fun.'

Little Elephant was very happy and loved his new slippers! He put them on just as the herd was about to get going. The ox-pecker settled on Little Elephant's back, and they happily went on their way.

Little Elephant did not whine any more and he did not tug on mommy's tail with his trunk. He walked proudly and sang with his family:

Elephants are we
Marching happily
We toot our song
As we go along
For elephants are we!

Little Elephant was so pleased with his new slippers that he thought up a new song to sing while walking:

Branches and leaves
For natural weaves.
We journey far and long
With slippers and a song!

'Story bones' – Hair-brushing story

At a workshop in Hong Kong, a mother of a two-and-a-half-year-old girl talked about her child's fussy behaviour around her hair … mainly that she would not let her mother brush or tie it up. As the child was quite young, the mother went back home and worked with some simple images in very simple story ways, adapting them to suit the hairstyle – from a pony to butterflies (see following email from the child's kindergarten teacher). There are a few story bones to work with here for children (girls) of many different ages!

Email from the teacher: ' … Since Cheuk Yin is very fond of horses, Fanny made up a story about a little horse that always wanted to run free in the field. The mother horse said it needed to tie up the hair into a ponytail in order to run freely, and so Cheuk Yin started coming to school with a ponytail. This is how she encouraged Cheuk Yin to comb and tie her hair. The next week, her mother wanted to tie her hair on both sides, so said they were going to make two little butterflies. It's not really a story but an image for her. But interestingly enough, when they went out this very morning, they started seeing butterflies around, and when they arrived at the field before reaching my kindergarten, they saw 20 to 30 butterflies flying … what a sight!' Both the butterfly and pony image helped the child accept having her mother tie up her hair.

12

Intolerance/Lack of Acceptance (of self and others)

Silvester the Snail
by Alfira Fisher

Note from the author: 'Silvester the Snail' was written for a five-year-old girl who loved animals. It aimed to help her find peace and self-acceptance within her family and to deal with the issue of sibling jealousy. It contains the seed that, through her own self-acceptance, she would be loved and supported for who she is. The story assisted healing dialogue to take place between family members. It is a story about acceptance of oneself.

Once upon a time, in a land where the mountains catch the clouds in the sky, there lived a tiny slow-moving creature called Silvester. Silvester was a forest snail. He lived under an old rotting log and ate many different kinds of fungi.

Silvester would wake up inside his shell every morning, and after a yawn and a slight wriggle he would pop his head out to see what kind of day it was and to watch his forest friends. Some days it was very quiet in the forest and he would stay inside his shell, warm and protected. On other days it was not so quiet. Silvester would watch his friends busy at work, moving quickly from place to place.
    'What an adventure everyone else is having,' he would say to himself! 'It seems I never get to go anywhere or do anything. And when I do get to go somewhere it takes me all day … O poor me!'

Suddenly Mr Bee buzzed merrily by and noticed that Silvester was feeling a little down. 'Hello Silvester', said Mr Bee. 'Hello,' said Silvester, 'what a busy bee you are, flying from flower to flower and going wherever you want.'

'Yes, I am very busy. I was just thinking how nice it is for you to move slowly and quietly through the day, and watch us all in our busy doings' said Mr Bee. 'Oh I didn't think about that', said Silvester. 'Yes, it does feel good to move slowly and quietly through the day.'

Then Mr Bee went on: 'How lucky you are to carry your home on your back.' Silvester replied, 'Yes, it is very quiet and cosy, and fits me perfectly.'

'How nice it must be to have that space all to yourself,' said Mr Bee. 'I share my home with all my brothers and sisters. It can be very crowded and noisy with everyone buzzing.'

'How different we both are', thought Silvester …

Just then, Mr Brush Turkey wandered up and overheard them talking. He told Silvester that sometimes he had to wander for hours before returning home in the evening, and when he did arrive home he would often find other forest animals sleeping in his nest.

'Oh,' said Silvester, 'I feel very lucky to carry my home on my back.' And he crawled back inside feeling very content. 'I am very happy to be me', he thought.

Seasons

A very simple story-rhyme for an older child to help accept a new baby in the house, and give a sense of the passing of time as related to the growth of little children. Parents could help the sibling make a book from this rhyme (with the child drawing the pictures). The idea for this was suggested at a workshop in Hobart. Note: This baby was born at the beginning of spring, hence the poem begins in spring. The words could be adapted to suit any time of year. It could also be extended with new aspects of a toddler's growth. The writing process might also be quite cathartic for the parent.

Baby came down to the world in the spring
Flowers opened their petals, the little birds sang.

In the summer the watermelon tasted so sweet
Baby licked a small piece, and loved the new treat.

In autumn the leaves tumbled down from the trees,
Baby sat on a blanket and watched them, so pleased.

The winter winds blew and we wrapped baby tight,
Brisk walks with the pram were a constant delight.

Then came the new spring, and baby stood tall,
First one step, then two – no longer so small!

Soon baby will play, with me and my ball!

Canoe Girl

In response to several emails (one from Ireland and one from California) with concerns about white-skinned children making fun of black-skinned children, I wrote the following story for two children aged four and six. I took the idea from the 'Cloud Boy' story that I had written for my own son (see Healing Stories for Challenging Behaviour*). This Canoe Girl story aims to help black children (living in a predominantly white community), who may complain about having black skin, or say they want to have a white body, develop a sense of their own identity.*

*   This story was written for use with some props – these could be as simple as a seedpod for the boat (or a small carved wooden canoe) and a little hand-made, dark-skinned doll. Note: In a predominantly black community, this story could be reversed for white children*

There was once a Canoe Girl who lived in a small wooden canoe on a long river that wound its way from one side of the land to the other. Canoe Girl slept each night in her canoe bed, rocked to sleep by the gentle river breezes. For breakfast she ate fruit that she gathered from the berry bushes on the riverbank, and in the evening she would catch and cook tasty fish for dinner. Canoe Girl had skin the brown of cocoa, hair and eyes the colour of the dark canoe wood, and wore a dress the red of the juicy berries she ate for breakfast.

For a long time, Canoe Girl was very happy living on the river all by herself. She loved floating downstream through the shady forests, riding the rapids through the mountain valleys, and racing with the wind that blew along the river as it crossed the sunny plains.

Sometimes the river passed through villages and towns, and Canoe Girl could see little children, just about her size, playing in the fields and the gardens near the riverbank. Then, within a few minutes, the river would take the boat onwards, leaving the playing children behind.

One day, the canoe was floating slowly through a town and came close to a sandy beach where children were digging in the sand and splashing in the water. Canoe Girl could see how much fun these children were having, and decided she wanted to leave her river home to play and live with other children. She pulled her canoe close to the riverbank and began to paddle slowly along the edge of the water, looking for a friend – one who would play with her and look after her ... but where could such a friend be found?

Note: After telling this story several times, a small dark-skinned doll and a canoe (made from a seedpod or carved wooden boat) could be given to the child as a present (perhaps they could find it by their bed when they wake in the morning). In the same way that my son found 'Cloud Boy' and immediately connected with it, this could help the child connect to her new, dark-skinned friend.

The Three Butterflies

A wonderful story for three- to five-year-olds for 'acceptance of differences' – contributed by Ellon Gold, Periwinkle Children's Centre, Byron Bay. Source of story unknown. It can be presented as a simple puppet show using little marionette butterflies made from felt or coloured fleece.

There were once three butterfly sisters, called Red Butterfly, Yellow Butterfly and Blue Butterfly. They would fly from flower to flower every day, collecting honey and pollen in the sunshine.

One day, as they were out in the sunshine, visiting the flowers, some rain clouds started to gather. The sky grew quite dark, until soon it started to rain and rain and rain. The three butterfly sisters were soon drenched with rain with their poor wings quite wet. As they were a long way from their home, they had to fly in the pouring rain to find some shelter together.

The three butterfly sisters flew to a red rose and said to the rose, 'Dear red rose, we are wet from the pouring rain. Could you please open your petals and let us in?'

The red rose said, 'Only red butterfly can come in as she is the same colour as me.'

The red butterfly said, 'If you will not let my sisters in, I would rather fly in the rain and find other shelter.'

So off they went again in the rain looking for a dry place to rest.

Soon the three butterfly sisters come upon a yellow daffodil and asked, 'Dear yellow daffodil, we are wet from the pouring rain. Could you please open your petals and let us in?'

The yellow daffodil said, 'Only yellow butterfly can come in as she is the same colour as me.'

The yellow butterfly said 'If you will not let my sisters in, I would rather fly in the rain and find other shelter.'

So again they went off in the rain.

After some time, the three butterfly sisters saw a bluebell flower. They flew over to it and asked,

'Dear bluebell, we are wet from the pouring rain. Could you please open your petals and let us in?'

The bluebell looked up and said, 'Only blue butterfly can come in as she is the same colour as me.'

The blue butterfly said, 'If you will not let my sisters in, I would rather fly in the rain and find other shelter.'

So they again went on, flying in the rain, looking for somewhere to dry their wings.

Now Father Sun, who had been watching from above, just behind the clouds, thought it was so lovely to see the three butterfly sisters always together and caring for each other. So Father Sun pushed the rain clouds away and he started to shine and shine and shine.

The sunshine helped to dry the butterflies' wet wings, and when the three butterfly sisters looked up to thank Father Sun they saw something beautiful. Stretched across the sky was a rainbow, with colours Red, Orange, Yellow, Green, Blue and Purple – all the colours altogether.

Father Sun had left a special gift in the sky, to remind everyone of how all the colours can live together happily.

The Rainbow Horses

An anti-discrimination story – which I wrote in the late 1990s for the children of the new South Africa (the 'Rainbow Nation'). Suitable for five- to ten-year-olds.

In the land where the rainbow ends, there once lived many horses; and each horse had a beautiful mane of a different colour. Their flowing colour manes were the prized possession of these horses, and because each horse was so proud of its chosen colour, they lived together only with others of the same, and wanted nothing to do with anyone else.

The purple horses lived in the mountains, the green ones lived in the forests, the red ones lived on the rocky plains, the blue ones lived by the river, the yellow ones lived on the coastline, and the orange ones lived in the desert.

For many years the horses had lived in their own colour groups, but there came a time when the younger horses longed to wander and explore the land. As they did so, the horses with different-coloured manes began to meet and mix with each other … and then fights would often break out to prove whose coloured silken manes were better and more beautiful than the rest.

Until this time, the golden sun had always shone brightly on the land where the rainbow ends, but now each new conflict between the horses created a new, tiny, grey cloud in the sky. At first these tiny, grey clouds could hardly be noticed – they were just dots in the blue sky. But as time went on and the different-coloured horses spread throughout the land, conflicts grew worse until the tiny grey clouds started to join together. At last, one day, the whole sky was full of great grey clouds.

Now the golden sun could no longer shine down on the land where the rainbow ends and the land grew very dark and cold. The grey clouds started to rain on the land; and it rained and rained for so many days that the rivers overflowed, and the plains and valleys were flooded with water.

As the water rose higher and higher, this forced all the horses of the land, of every colour, to retreat to the high slopes of the tallest mountain in the centre of the plains. This great mountain was so high and cold that no grasses grew here and the sides were very rocky. There was nothing to eat so the horses grew very hungry and weak, and began to huddle together in the rocky caves just to keep warm. Because keeping warm was now so important, it didn't seem to matter what colour of mane each horse possessed, and the conflicts slowly calmed then stopped.

At the same time that the conflicts ended, the rains also stopped. A gap appeared in the dark clouds above the rocky mountain slopes, and a ray of sunlight shone through. In this ray of light a shining angel appeared, and slowly descended on the golden beams to a slope close to where the horses were sheltering from the cold. As the angel came to rest on the ground, the horses could see that she was holding a golden loom in her arms. She put the loom down beside her and spoke to them:

I have come from the Sun King with a message of help. In his garden in heaven there lives a golden horse and this golden horse has the power to bring light back to your land and rid your sky of these dark clouds. But for it to journey from its heavenly garden down to your land, it needs a pair of wings, and these wings must come from you. On my golden weaving loom I can weave such a pair of wings, but I will need the silken hair from all your silken manes for the threads.

Now this was a very difficult request. All the horses had been so proud of their beautiful, coloured manes. But they knew there was no other way! So one by one, they stepped up to the angel and bowed their heads, allowing their silken manes to be shorn off. When all the horses had taken their turn, a great pile of coloured, silken threads lay upon the ground. Then they watched as the angel sat at her loom and started to weave from side to side, backwards and forwards, side to side, backwards and forwards, side to side, backwards and forwards … until a pair of beautiful rainbow wings lay stretched across the loom.

Taking the silken wings carefully in her arms, the angel rose up again on a ray of light and disappeared back through the gap in the dark clouds. She journeyed with the wings all the way to the Sun King's heavenly garden;' and there she attached them to the golden horse. The winged golden horse then flew up and out of the garden and across the sky, down to the land where the rainbow ends. His golden light was so bright that the grey clouds scattered in his path, and the waters flooding the land dried up.

Now the horses could go back to their homes and once more live in warmth together and find food to eat. In giving up their silken, coloured manes they had overcome their vanity and pride, and now they could easily live in harmony. Peace once again reigned over the land.

As for the winged golden horse, he made his home at the foot of the rainbow. To this day he has lived on in our world, ready to be there when needed to drive away any dark clouds that try to hide the golden light of the sun.

The Little Drummer Boy

This Christmas story is a wonderful example of accepting each other's qualities, and understanding that we all have different kinds of gifts to give. It was inspired by two different children's carols – 'I said the donkey, all shaggy and brown' and 'The Drummer Boy'. It is hard to put an age grouping to this story. I have used it with four- to eight-year-olds but its Christmas theme could be for any age.

Long, long ago, in a land far across the sea, a new baby king was born into the world.

This baby king was so special that over the roof where he was born there shone a brilliant star, and wise men came to visit him, travelling from afar. This baby king was so special that all of heaven's angels in their glory filled the sky to sing his story. This baby king was so special that animals and shepherds came to bring their humble gifts, and cuckoos, doves and pigeons sang his praises.

Out on the hillside a little shepherd boy was sitting in the fields and listening to his animal friends talking excitedly to each other. They were talking of the new baby king who had just been born in the town below. They were sharing the news of the gifts they wished to give to this new king:

'I carried his mother all the way to Bethlehem town,' said the donkey all shaggy and brown.

'I gave him my manger for his bed,' said the cow all white and red.

'I gave him my wool to keep him warm,' said the sheep with the curly horn.

'We cooed him to sleep so he would not cry,' said the dove, 'my mate and I.'

Then the friends turned to the little shepherd boy, and asked:

'What gift can you bring, to the baby king?'

The shepherd boy replied: 'I am just a poor child, I have no gift to bring. What gift can a poor child bring to a baby king?'

It was now getting dark, and his friends made their way back to the farm. Only the little shepherd boy stayed to watch over his goats who always stayed longer to eat more grass on the hillside.

Soon it was time even for the goats to return to the farm, and the little shepherd boy started to play his drum to call the goats in, one by one.

Pa-rum pum-pum pum, Rum-pum pum-pum, Rum-pum pum-pum.

For every goat he had a different tune to play on his drum, and slowly the goats heard their tune and followed him home, in a long line, one by one.

Pa-rum pum-pum pum, Rum-pum pum-pum, Rum-pum pum-pum.

That night, lying in his bed, the little shepherd boy couldn't sleep – he was thinking about the new baby king, and wondering what gift a poor boy could bring to a little king.

Then he had an idea – he could play his drum for the new baby king!

He was so excited with his idea that he climbed out of bed, picked up his drum and set off down the road and into the town, searching, searching for the stable where he had been told the little king was sleeping.

'I must play my drum very softly for this little one,' he thought, 'so softly that it will help him to sleep, not wake him up!'

And so he stood by the stable door, and played a soft tune, under the bright stars and the shining moon:

> *Baby Jesus, pa-rum pum-pum pum,*
> *I am a poor child too, pa-rum pum-pum pum,*
> *I have no gift to bring, pa-rum pum-pum pum,*
> *That's fit to give a king, pa-rum pum-pum pum,*
> *Rum-pum pum-pum, Rum-pum pum-pum,*
> *Shall I play for you, pa-rum pum-pum pum,*
> *On my drum?*

Mother Mary was cradling the little baby in her arms, and smiled a thank-you to the little shepherd boy when he had finished playing. And the shepherd boy was sure he saw the little king smile to him from his deep sleep in his mother's arms.

The little shepherd boy was so happy. He set off for home, playing his drum and singing the whole way along the road and back to his house.

The shining stars looked down from above, and twinkled even brighter that night, the night the little shepherd boy brought his special gift of music to the new baby king.

> *Baby Jesus, pa-rum pum-pum pum,*
> *I am a poor child too, pa-rum pum-pum pum,*
> *I have no gift to bring, pa-rum pum-pum pum,*
> *That's fit to give a king, pa-rum pum-pum pum,*
> *Rum-pum pum-pum, Rum-pum pum-pum,*
> *Shall I play for you, pa-rum pum-pum pum,*
> *On my drum?*

'Story bones' – The Sled Race and other ideas

The idea of a team of husky dogs pulling a sled, or a team of horses pulling a carriage, was used by several different groups for similar challenging situations involving 5–10-year-old children with low self-esteem, withdrawn and lacking confidence and not accepted by the group. This was a common theme at workshops on three different continents – Asia, Africa and America!

I have included the 'bones' of three story ideas below.

The Sled Race

Drum song to start and end the race – husky team (with shy dog given an 'Inuit' name) – team starts off happy then meets obstacles – deep crevices, and a storm, and the team loses its way – the shy dog helps the team – teaches them how to build snow houses to keep warm, then read the stars to find the way home – the shy dog uses 'Inuit' knowledge and saves the team.

The Husky Team and the St Bernard

The husky team sets off on a journey pulling a sled – a St Bernard dog wants to join the team but all the husky dogs laugh at this dog – it is a different colour and shape and size – they do not want him in the team – team sets off, laughing at the dog they had left behind – not long after setting out they get stuck in a crevice – the St Bernard dog comes to the rescue and pulls them out.

The Gypsy Wagon

A team of four draft horses is pulling a gypsy wagon – the wagon is carrying a mother, father and a little child through the mountains – one of the horses is not as strong and big as the other three and the wagon driver keeps shouting at the weaker horse – they reach a river that is too deep to cross. The smaller weaker horse turns out to be the strongest swimmer, and swims across to the other bank, firstly carrying the mother and child, then the father, with a rope to pull all the heavy items from the wagon across the water, then finally the wagon is floated across and the other three horses are helped to get across too.

13

Lack of Confidence/Resilience

The Winged Horse

This story was written as a resilience-building, motivational story for primary schoolchildren. A colleague recently used it with her class of 10-year-olds, with a particular boy in mind who needed help to strengthen his will to do things, and his general lack of interest in life. This boy listened intently from start to finish then put up his hand to make a comment – 'I think the boy should conquer the quests, not "complete" the quests'. The teacher was most impressed with his enthusiastic engagement with the story, as this was not a common experience. His suggestion seemed to work so well that I have now changed the verse to include 'conquer'.

There was once a boy who wanted a horse more than anything else in the whole world!

But he didn't just want an ordinary horse. The boy wished for a horse that could fly: he wanted to ride a winged horse!

When he told his friends of his wish, they all laughed at him and told him there was no such thing in the world. But the boy knew that there *was* such a thing – he was sure he had seen it flying across the night sky and disappearing up into the great mountains. One day he talked to his father about this, and his father smiled a deep smile. 'I remember that a wise teacher from long ago told me stories of such a horse', he said. 'Why don't you go and visit her, and she may be able to help your wish come true.'

The boy's father told him where his old teacher now lived. Her home was in the middle of the forest between the town and the great mountains. So the next day, the boy packed some food in his backpack and set out on the long journey. After many hours of walking, he finally reached a little cabin in a clearing where the sunlight was shining down its golden rays through the dark green trees. On the verandah of the cabin sat a beautiful old woman with long, silver hair and twinkling eyes. The boy introduced himself and gave greetings from his father. Then he told the old woman of his wish to ride on a winged horse.

The old woman took some time to answer, and finally she told him that, yes, she knew where the winged horse lived, but its home was high up in a cave on the great mountains where no man had ever been able to climb before. And even if someone could reach the cave, guarding its entrance was a vicious dragon that would be impossible to pass. And even if someone could find a way to get past the dragon, the winged horse was so shy of humans that it would be difficult to coax him out of the cave – unless, she whispered, you waited until the moon was full. On full-moon nights the horse loved to come out into the silver light and fly across the sky.

The old women invited the boy to stay the night in her cabin; and the next morning, after a nourishing breakfast of eggs and honey cakes, she gave the boy three things to help him on his quest – a sharp metal knife, a wooden flute and a strand of her long, silver hair.

'These may help you to find your way where no other person has dared to go', she told him. The boy tied the silver strand of hair around his neck, put the knife and flute in his pack, and thanked the old woman. As he turned to go, she called out to him, 'Whenever you reach a difficult turn on your road, remember to say to yourself:

With my head, heart and hands, I will do my best;
With my head, heart and hands, I will conquer my quest!

Feeling encouraged by these words, the boy continued along the path that led out of the other side of the forest and towards the great mountains.

After walking for many hours, he finally came to a place where the foothills of the mountains met the sheer cliffs towering to the sky. The steep walls seemed too sheer to climb. The boy sat at the bottom, and remembering the old woman's advice, said to himself:

With my head, heart and hands, I will do my best;
With my head, heart and hands, I will conquer my quest!

Then he noticed the strong vines growing in the trees near where he was sitting, and he had an idea. With the knife that the old woman had given to him, and his strong and nimble hands, he started to cut the vines and weave and knot a rope ladder. When the ladder was ready, he stood back far enough and threw a vine up to hook onto a strong tree growing from the top of the cliffs. Then he was able to hoist the ladder and climb up, rung by rung, slowly and carefully, until he reached the top.

At the top of the cliffs, just as the old woman had said, there was a vicious dragon guarding the entrance of a cave. The dragon was the most frightening creature that the boy had ever imagined and it seemed impossible to pass – its great head was high in the air and spitting and striking out towards him.

Keeping a safe distance, the boy sat down on the edge of the cliffs to think about what to do. Then he remembered the old woman's advice:

With my head, heart and hands, I will do my best;
With my head, heart and hands, I will conquer my quest!

Suddenly he had an idea. Taking the flute out of his backpack, he started to play a most beautiful tune. He kept on playing with all his heart, and after a long time, he started to notice that the dragon had stopped spitting and striking out towards him, and instead was dancing a slow dance, first with just his head and then his whole body. The boy kept on playing and eventually the dragon grew so tired from his dancing that he put his head down to rest on his great scaly body and fell fast asleep.

The boy put his flute back in his pack, and crept past the sleeping dragon to the entrance of the cave. He peered inside. The cave was black as darkest night, and the boy could neither see nor hear any sign of the winged horse he was hoping to now meet.

He stood in the blackness and tried to think about what to do. Then once again he remembered the old woman's advice:

With my head, heart and hands, I will do my best;
With my head, heart and hands, I will conquer my quest!

So far he had used his hands to make the strong ladder to scale the cliffs. And he had played the music to tame the dragon with all his heart. So now it was time to think up a clever plan to coax the winged horse (if he was really inside the cave) to come out to meet him.

Then he noticed something softly shining in the darkness. He looked down and realized it was the strand of silver hair that he had tied around his neck. He lifted it over his head and held it out so that it made a shining silver loop in front of him – didn't the old woman tell him that the winged horse loved silver light!

He turned to go back to the entrance, thinking he would wait there with his silver loop, that he had now decided could easily be used like a bridle. And with the good fortune that seemed to be with him on this quest, he noticed that outside the cave the daylight was fading and the full moon was rising over the edge of the cliffs. The full moon shone into the cave, turning the blackness into silver light. And standing deep inside was the beautiful winged horse!

Holding the silver bridle at the opening of the cave, the boy stood patiently and confidently, and started to softly sing:

> Winged horse, come to me, I will be your friend – trust me!
> Together we can ride the sky, together we can fly up high!

After some time, the horse slowly moved forward, came close to the boy and nuzzled his head into the boy's chest. The boy softly stroked his long mane that was shining with rainbow colours in the moonlight. Then the boy slipped the silver bridle over the horse's head, softly singing all the while:

> Winged horse, come to me, I will be your friend – trust me!
> Together we can ride the sky, together we can fly up high!

When the boy felt confident that the horse knew he had found a friend he could trust, the boy carefully climbed up on his shining white back, and took hold of the silver bridle. The horse then spread its wings and took off from the cliff tops. Up, up, up, it flew, until the boy and the horse were riding across the night sky with the clouds and the stars and the silver moon.

All night the horse flew the boy through the sky, and then as dawn grew pale in the east, the horse landed down by the boy's home, right outside his bedroom window.

'Keep the silver bridle,' the horse whispered to the boy, 'and every full moon I will come back to collect you so together we can go riding across the night sky.'

The horse bent his head down and the boy slipped off the silver bridle, put it back around his neck, and climbed through his window and into his warm, waiting bed.

The boy slept a very long time and his dreams were of travels to beautiful lands.

He awoke to find his father sitting by his bed and holding his hand. 'My wish has come true,' said the boy to his father, 'and every full moon I will ride a winged horse across the sky.'

His father smiled a knowing smile, then went into the kitchen to make a breakfast of eggs and honey cakes. His son had been on a great journey and now would be very hungry!

The Gnomes and the Golden Crowns
by Silviah Njagi and Susan Perrow

The initial idea for this story came in response to an early morning robbery in a school in Nairobi, a few hours before the children arrived for class. The school office and part of the kindergarten were vandalized, so the children were kept outside all morning to protect them from the shock of seeing their room in chaos. In the afternoon, most of the damage was repaired while the children were safely at home. In the days ahead, stronger steel doors and windows were put in. Their teacher, Silviah Njagi, had a clear aim – she wanted a story that, in her words, 'was really about us and what we could do to help ourselves, as opposed to focusing on the thieves, whom iron bars can't stop anyway!' (An unfortunate fact of life in Kenya!) Silviah thought that the important resolution for a healing story was how the parents, the children and the teachers could work together in rebuilding the kindergarten, giving them courage and confidence to face the future no matter what obstacles may appear!

Through email dialogue, I worked with Silviah to produce the final version that involved the little gnomes making golden crowns. Silviah's initial idea was to have them making golden swords, but we decided that we really didn't want the children to get attached to a weapon – is fighting the way forward? The crown gives each little gnome a light, a new courage, a new strength, to carry with them everywhere they go. Also in a practical sense, the light of the crown becomes like a miner's light, and seemed a better fit for Silviah's choice of storyline. We discussed what should happen to the giant, but decided that we couldn't promise the thieves wouldn't return, so it seemed best to leave this unresolved, and focus on building confidence and resilience instead. The story used images from local surroundings – described as follows by Silviah: 'Our kindergarten is surrounded by tall jacaranda trees which begin to bloom in September, and burst open fully in October. The garden has slopes that form little mountains, and dragonflies flit around in anticipation of the short rains in mid-October ... '

Once upon a time in a land where the tall jacaranda bloomed, there was a big mountain. Inside this mountain lived a family of gnomes in a rock-cave home.

Early in the morning the gnomes would wake up, put their sacks upon their backs and their little hammers upon their shoulders. Together they would march down, deeper and deeper, into the tunnels of the mountain to dig for treasure. With their hammers they would knock against the solid rock and there they would find gold. Then they would take the golden rock and rub-a-dub at the gold until it shone brighter than the sun itself.

At the end of the day the little gnomes would carry the gold back to their cave and store it in a clear glass jar. The golden jar filled the cave home with a warming light.

The good work of the gnomes continued for a long time. But one morning, something changed. In the distant valley there lived a needy, greedy giant who slept most of the time unless he was out stealing treasures from others. For quite some time he had known about the mountain gnomes ... how hard they worked and how bright their gold shone. The needy greedy giant loved gold.

So on a particular morning, the needy greedy giant decided to visit the gnomes' cave and steal the gold for himself. The giant listened to hear the feet of the gnomes marching deeper and deeper into the mountain. As soon as he heard their hammers clack, clack, clack, he crept into the cave and stole all the gold out of the glass jar. He then ran as fast as his giant legs would carry him until he came back to his valley.

When the gnomes came home in the evening they were shocked to find their cave so dark. Immediately they knew that their gold had been stolen. They put the gold that they had found on that day into the glass jar but it was only a little, so it did not shine as bright. The gnomes huddled together, wishing they could find a way to make the golden light shine brighter.

A dragonfly flitting outside the cave, heard the gnomes' wish and sang a song into their dreams that night:

With the little gold you have, make golden crowns so bright,
Wear them everywhere you go, to light the darkest night.

The next morning when the gnomes woke up, they remembered the song of the dragonfly. Together they collected some wood and made a fire. With this they melted the small amount of gold and beat it into thin strips and shaped it to make little crowns for each and every one of them. As they worked they sang:

With the little gold we have, we are making crowns so bright,
To wear them everywhere we go, to light the darkest night.

When they finished their work, the little crowns shone brightly. The gnomes wore them on their heads and they felt stronger and braver. They now had the courage to march deeper and deeper into the tunnels of the mountain with their sacks upon their backs, their little hammers upon their shoulders and their golden crowns lighting the way.

From that time on, the gnomes continued working hard. They found more gold and put it in their glass jar to light up their cave home. They always wore their golden crowns to help light up the dark tunnels under the mountain, as they happily sang and worked together each day.

With the little gold we have, we are making crowns so bright,
To wear them everywhere we go, to light the darkest night.

The Little Pigs and the Hyena

A Kenyan version of the classic tale of The Three Little Pigs. An enduring story that emphasizes the importance of strong foundations and resilience for overcoming obstacles. I have re-written it as a morning story ring (in song and rhyme and movement). This is my favourite way of sharing this story with children aged from three to six years. Working with this particular storyline in movement seems a very appropriate (and thera- peutic) way to help children through the strong journey – they always love finishing with the 'brick-on-stone' song and shaking their fingers at the evil hyena that has been finally overcome! Of course, a similar version could be told using the original wolf character.

Song: The first little pig left home one day, and met a man upon his way (2×)

Verse: The man gave the first little pig some straw to build his house.

Song: *Build your house up, build it high,*
       Point the chimney to the sky,
       See the roof and see the floor,
       See the shining little golden door.

Verse: When the house of straw was finished the little pig climbed inside. Then the hyena came along and BLEW that house of straw far and wide!

'I'll huff and I'll puff and I'll BLOW your house down!' (3×)

Song: *The second little pig left home one day, and met a man upon his way.* (2×)

Verse: The man gave the second little pig some sticks to build his house.

Song: *Build your house up, build it high,*
       Point the chimney to the sky,
       See the roof and see the floor,
       See the shining little golden door.

Verse: When the house of sticks was finished the little pig climbed inside. Then the hyena came along and BLEW that house of sticks far and wide!

'I'll huff and I'll puff and I'll BLOW your house down!' (3×)

Song: *The third little pig left home one day, and met a man upon his way.* (2×)

Verse: The man gave the third little pig some bricks to build his house.
       The third little pig worked hard and long, to build his house of bricks so true and strong.

Song: *Build your house up, build it high,*
       Point the chimney to the sky,
       See the roof and see the floor,
       See the shining little golden door.

Verse: When the house of bricks was finished the little pig climbed inside. Then the hyena came along – but no matter how hard the hyena BLEW and BLEW and BLEW and BLEW and BLEW – he could not blow down that house of bricks so strong and true!

And so the hyena had to go away – and come back with a different plan the next day …

Song:
Dig, dig, diggety dig, meet me in the morning, little pig,
At Farmer Shamba a turnip to dig – soup for you and me!
Shake, shake, shakety shee, in the orchard we'll climb the tree,
Apples ripe and red we'll see – in the morning early.
Roly-poly tumble-bumble, what is this I hear a-rumble?
From the market and down the hill – then it stops! – and all is still!

Verse: Hyena tried this trick and that, but could not catch
The third little pig in his house of bricks – much
stronger than the straw or sticks!
And so, up onto the roof the hyena did go,
And down the chimney with a hey and a ho –
Right into the hot pot on the stove below –
With a hey, and a hi, and a ho, with a hey, and a hi, and a ho!

Song: *Brick on stone for piggies' home, Build it as strong as can be!*
Hyena ho I'm laughing so – You'll never, never, never catch me!

The Shining Star
by Rosalind Veness

Note from the author: The grandmother of one of my students, an 8-year-old boy, recently gave me some important feedback. She said her grandson was concerned about why he is having remedial help, asking 'Is there something wrong with me?' I felt the best way to address this lack of confidence was to use a story. I have used the metaphor of a star, because all my students are shining stars, but sometimes they just need a little bit of extra 'polish'. I wanted to reflect the fact that it is the student who does the hard work, with a bit of help from the practitioner. The story didn't connect with the boy I thought I had written it for, but it did seem to help another child (girl aged 9). She was restless, verging on hyperactivity, and had difficulty in forming friendships. She enjoyed the story, connected with the story, and later told me, 'I saw that star.'

Have you ever sat outside at night and looked up at the stars? Perhaps you wondered how they came to be shining so brightly.

Once there was a little star who felt a bit dull. He struggled to show his light, wanting to be able to shine more brightly, and bring more light into the world. He was worried that even though he always tried very hard, the children down on earth might not think his light was bright enough.

So, he closed his eyes and made a big wish.

Then his fairy godmother appeared, and waved her magic wand. She gave the little star a tiny bag of magic stardust to help him shine.

So the little star used the magic stardust to polish himself all over. His starry points spread out in many directions. It was very hard work, doing all that polishing, and he had so many points to cover, but he kept going because he really wanted to shine a special light into the world.

He wanted to keep the magic stardust and his polishing as a special secret, so he didn't tell the other stars what he was doing, and worked away quietly when none of the other stars were watching.

Every day his light shone a little brighter. Now this little star is one of the brightest shining stars in the sky.

Perhaps you will see him, next time you go outside at night, shining brightly and lighting up the world.

Little Gold Horse

An autumn/Easter story for four- to six-year-olds to help with building confidence and overcoming fear. The story was inspired by the golden cassia flowers that blossom in the autumn in the gardens and bush-land around my home on the east coast of NSW – flowers that are forever connected in my memory with Easter time in Australia.

There was once a Little Gold Horse,

> *Galloping ho, galloping ho, galloping galloping galloping ho*

He lived in the garden of the Sun King's palace, high up in the sky, and all day long he would run wild and free amongst the snowy clouds and across the bright blue sky.

> *Galloping ho, galloping ho, galloping galloping galloping ho*

One day the Sun King called Little Gold Horse to him and said …

'Little Gold Horse, for a long time you have been running wild and free in my garden and I have been watching you every year grow bigger and stronger, stronger and bigger. Now that you are big enough and strong enough it is time for you to leave my garden and travel as a messenger to a world far away. I have gifts of sun gold for you to take there, but beware, there may be danger on the way!'

And so, with the gifts of sun gold on his back, the Little Gold Horse left the Sun King's garden and set out on his long journey across the sky.

Galloping ho, galloping ho, galloping galloping galloping ho

It was not long before the snow white clouds grew darker and darker, and suddenly the Little Gold Horse found himself in the Land of Storms. Cloud mountains towered over him on every side! He could hear thunder and see lightning in the distance, and the wind was blowing so strongly it was hard for him to move forward. However, he struggled on …

Galloping ho, galloping ho, galloping galloping galloping ho (very slowly)

The noise of thunder grew louder and louder, and the flash of lightning brighter and brighter. Just when the wind grew so strong that Little Gold Horse could move forward no more, he found himself on the banks of Wild Storm River. Here the thunder was louder than the sound of a thousand marching giants, and the lightning flashes were so bright that Little Gold Horse had to close his eyes and turn away.

How was he going to cross Wild Storm River? How was he going to take the gifts of sun gold to the world on the other side?

Just then, there was a flash of bright colour amongst the dark clouds, and seven winged horses came galloping past Little Gold Horse:

Rainbow horses galloping by, spreading their wings across the sky
A rainbow bridge to make, hey-ho, a-galloping galloping galloping go.

The winged horses came to Wild Storm River and spread their rainbow wings to form a wide bridge for Little Gold Horse to cross over. Up, up, up he climbed, and down, down, down, until he was safely across Wild Storm River. On the other side, the cloud mountains grew smaller and smaller until the sky was clear and blue. Little Gold Horse could see the forests and valleys and plains in the world below. He turned to wave a thank-you to the rainbow horses, but they had already disappeared back behind the land of storms.

And so he kept on his way,

Galloping ho, galloping ho, galloping galloping galloping ho

When he reached the world below he began to gallop across the plains and through the forests, once again wild and free. As he galloped along, he left his gifts of sun gold on many of the bushes and many of the trees for the people of this world to find and share.

And at the Easter time of year, you may see that the Little Gold Horse has come to visit some trees near you and left some Easter gold for you to find and share with your family and friends.

The Light of the Future

A midwinter festival story written for six- to ten-year-olds (and adults!) and used at a community festival celebrating the theme of finding 'light' and overcoming fear in the darkest and longest night of the year. It was told to a hundred parents and children (warmly wrapped up in coats and blankets) sitting under the great fig tree in the town park (I stood high up on the raised tree roots to tell the story). The storytelling was followed by a lantern walk along the winding path by the river. The path had recently been decorated with dreamtime drawings of different animals by local indigenous artists, and the children had made blue, yellow and red lanterns to carry on the lantern walk. It was a most empowering experience for young and old alike, and set the theme for many discussions both at home and at school.

Once upon a time it happened – where did it happen? Or, we might ask, where did it not happen? – there was a town in a valley filled with people who were peaceful and happy. Their children were healthy and happy, many beautiful flowers and fruits grew in their gardens, and the sun seemed to shine on their lives most of the time.

However, once a year, in the cold winter months, something happened that filled the people's hearts with fear. This was when the dragon, who lived in a dark cave in the mountains, woke up from his long sleep and set out on his slow journey down through the forests and fields towards the town. Now this was no ordinary dragon – he breathed blue, flickering flames and liked only the dark and cold. When he left his cave home each winter he would wrap himself in a dark swirl of mist and rain. As he journeyed down the valley he would leave a devastated trail of trees, plants and animals turned cold and lifeless by his breath of blue flames.

It was usually in the darkest winter nights that the dragon would set out hungrily on his journey. But every year the people would prepare for his attack by calling on the star spirits to bring down their bright light to guard the town. And every year the star spirits would come down in the depths of midwinter and shine their bright light over the town, forcing the dragon to turn back again, away from the light he hated so much, and retreat to the shelter of his dark cave.

For many, many years this happened; and over time the dragon grew angrier and angrier, and hungrier and hungrier. Wrapped in his swirls of mist and rain, each winter he ravaged the forests and countryside and laid waste to it more and more. But whenever he came close to the town the people could trust that the star spirits would come down and protect them with their bright, shining light.

Then one year, just after the star spirits had been to visit in the deep midwinter, and the dragon had once again been forced to return, angry and hungry, to his dark cave to sleep, the star spirits said to the people: 'We will not be coming back again – it is time that you find a way to visit us instead. We have star gifts in our star castle to give you, and these star gifts will protect you from the dragon.'

'But', the people cried, 'how can we find the way from our world up to the sky? How can we find the pathway that leads to the Star Castle?'

'With this we cannot help you', the star spirits replied, 'but when you come, our star gifts will be waiting for you.' And so saying, the star spirits returned to their home in the night sky, leaving the people wondering what to do.

'We must ask the oldest and wisest friend in the valley to help us', they all agreed. And so, the next day, leaving their children to play in their gardens, the people went to the edge of town where the great tree grew by the river. For this was the home of the tree spirit, oldest and wisest of all in the valley.

'Oh great tree spirit,' the people cried, 'we have come to you for help. Can you show us the way from our world up to the sky? We must visit the Star Castle and bring back the star gifts to protect our town from the dragon that will wake in the cold of next winter.'

There was a rustling of leaves and a shimmering of green gold. High up in the branches the tree spirit appeared and spoke to the people with a voice like the gentle wind: 'Yes, I can help you. I will lend you a special lantern to show you the way.' And the tree spirit floated down and disappeared between the roots of the trees, to return almost instantly with a shining crystal in her hands.

'This lantern', she said, 'I have taken from a crystal cave deep under the roots of my home. It is called 'The Light of the Future' and only when it is held by someone whose heart knows no fear will it light up and shine to show the way from this world up to the sky. Now, who will come forward to carry the lantern?'

The tree spirit then passed 'The Light of the Future' to the first of the townspeople who stepped forward, a man known to be one of the bravest and strongest of them all. But the moment it touched his hands 'The Light of the Future' stopped shining. He then passed it to the next person and the next and the next, until all the men and women of the town had had a turn at holding the crystal lantern – and not one of them could make it shine.

'Is there not one amongst you with no fear in your heart?' the tree spirit asked.

And then a small voice was heard to say: 'Let me try!'

The people looked down and there, standing with his eyes closed and hands outstretched, was a little blind child. He had not been left to play with all the other children. Because he could not see, his parents had to hold him by the hand and lead him everywhere they went.

'You,' the people laughed, 'but you cannot even see your way through your own town. How could you find the way from the world up to the sky?'

But the tree spirit had already placed the crystal lantern into the child's outstretched hands, and 'The Light of the Future' shone as brightly as the day. The face of the little child was shining too, because it seemed that suddenly he could see with eyes he had never used before. And the lantern was showing him a path that no one else could see. The child started to follow this new path, past the trees and over the bridge, until he disappeared from sight.

The townsfolk watched all this in great surprise, and when the child's parents tried to run after him, the tree spirit stood in their way. 'Let him go,' she said, 'you must trust in "The Light of the Future" and in your child's heart that has no fear. He will be back next winter with the star gifts you need to protect your town. Go home and watch each evening – soon you will see him as he journeys the starry zodiac path that stretches across the night sky.'

So the people returned to their homes and every evening they watched for signs of the child's journey from the world up to the sky. And soon, just as the tree spirit had said, they could see a glowing light, like a new star, moving slowly along the zodiac pathway that stretches across the night sky. All through the spring and into the summer they watched this light on its long journey, and then on midsummer's night it disappeared.

Then the next night the bright star reappeared with three new stars, twinkling blue, yellow and red. Together they started to move back slowly along the starry pathway and across the autumn sky.

Meanwhile, down in the town and the valley, the cold winds of winter began to blow. There was a rumbling and a shaking in the mountains as the dragon was heard to wake up in his dark cave. Wrapped in dark swirls of mist and rain that hid his monstrous shape, he began his long slow journey down the valley. Through the cold winter nights he moved, ravaging the forests and fields with his blue fiery breath, on his way towards the town.

The townspeople once again grew afraid – what if the child didn't return in time with the star gifts needed to protect their town? They trembled with fear for their own and their children's safety.

The days grew colder and colder, the nights darker and longer, and the dragon moved slowly towards the town. The people could now feel his breath of cold fire like a fierce wind blowing down the valley. Soon a dark mist settled over the land and the people huddled together in their homes, afraid to venture outdoors in the night.

Then came the shortest day of winter! As the people in their fear met together under the great tree to ask the tree spirit once more for help, they saw through the grey mists a flickering of bright lights. As they watched, the lights grew brighter – shining out, blue, yellow and red – and then the little child appeared, striding joyfully across the bridge and towards the tree. On his forehead he wore a shining blue star, over his heart was a radiant yellow star, and in the palm of his hand was a flaming red star. And in his other hand he carried the shining crystal lantern.

Waiting in the branches of the tree was the great tree spirit. She carefully reached down and lifted the star gifts from the little child and then hung them high up in the tree. Their light shone out brightly across the town, blue, yellow and red. Their light shone through the dark swirling mists and right into the eyes of the dragon who had just then reached the outer edge of the town. He gave a great cry as the bright lights blinded him, then he turned back into the mists and groped and stumbled his way back to his dark cave as fast as his monstrous dragon legs could carry him.

The tree spirit then took 'The Light of the Future', thanked the little child, and disappeared down through the roots of the tree to place it back in its crystal cave deep underground.

The people, led triumphantly by the little child who was once blind but could now see, returned to their homes for great feasting and celebration. That night they slept peacefully and unafraid. And the star gifts, blue, yellow and red, shone out brightly above the town, filling the winter's night with their radiant light.

And as far as I know, they are shining there still.

Ariadne's Thread – stories, crafts and 'maze' games

Stories, crafts and 'maze' games on the theme of 'finding one's way' and strengthening threads in one's life. Used in conjunction with the story of Ariadne's Thread (see below) with great success for three different groups of challenging 8–10-year-olds at a foster-children's camp called Camp Resilience, Lennox Head, NSW. There were 12 children in each group, mostly boys. All three groups of children (whom I had been warned could be very restless and uncooperative) were taken in by the imaginative approach and responded with excitement, enjoyment and concentration.

Relay Maze Game (helping to set the 'maze' theme through movement and activity)

- Working in pairs (go round group and call out numbers 1 – 6 twice, then ask the child to pair up with their matching number).
- Ask for all the pairs to line up along the wall, sitting on chairs.
- One partner runs to the end of the room to collect two pens and return them to the chairs.
- The next partner runs to the end of the room to collect 2 papers (printed with a maze puzzle) and return them.
- Both then kneel down and lean on the chairs to complete the puzzles.
- The first to finish the maze helps their partner, then both put up their hands. Points scored for 1st, 2nd and 3rd places.

Maze and Treasure Game

- Chairs back in circle ready to play *Maze and Treasure Game*
- Tell Maze and Treasure Story (see below).

Maze and Treasure Story

Imagine a great mountain, taller and greater than you have ever seen; and so huge that it can be seen from all across the land. Deep inside this mountain, at the end of many long passageways and tunnels, there is a cave. The passages and tunnels twist in and out (just like the maze you did this morning) and there are many false paths going to dead-ends. Some of the dead-ends are walls of rock that block the way; others are truly 'dead-ends' as they have gaping holes: if you fell into them you would be dead! There are many choices to make on this pathway, and there is only one right way to the cave. And as in all underground tunnels and passages, there is little or no light to show the way.

Inside the cave is a very large treasure box containing the most precious thing you could ever imagine owning in your whole life (I will leave it up to you to decide what your treasure is … it could be gold or diamonds, a favourite animal, a friend or family member whom you haven't seen for a long time, the rarest flower in the world … and when you decide what it is, you have to keep this a secret till the end of the session.)

You have rounded up two friends to help you travel the maze inside the mountain to reach the cave, get the treasure box and carry it out to safety.

Before you set out on this difficult journey (quest), you have to decide what you need to take with you to help you succeed. You are only allowed three things (one for each of you to carry).

- After telling the above story, divide the group of twelve into four lots of threes.
- In each group, negotiate four things you can take on the quest.
- Rejoin the whole group and share your four choices!

Now tell the following story …

Ariadne's Thread

(Note – this is a simplified version, deliberately kept short because of the poor concentration span of this particular group of foster children – a longer version could spend more time describing the battle between the Minotaur and Theseus and, if the group was aged 10 and over, continue on to include the more tragic ending relating to the death of Theseus' father).

There was once a king who ruled over a large island off the coast of Greece. He should have been a happy man, but his son had just been killed in battle by soldiers from a city in a land across the sea. The city was called Athens and the soldiers were called Athenians.

On hearing this terrible news, the king was so upset and angry that he sent a fleet of ships to attack and conquer Athens. Then he devised a plan that would exact revenge upon the Athenians.

Firstly he had his master-builder construct a maze, a house of winding passages. He built such a confusing maze that it quite deceived the eye with the conflicting puzzle of various wandering paths and dead-ends. So deceptive was the design that even the builder who had designed the maze was barely able to return to the entrance when he tried to navigate his way through.

In the centre of the maze the king kept a hideous creature on a long chain. It was called the Minotaur, the bull-man – half man and half bull. It had the head of a bull and the body of a man, and it lived off human flesh.

The king then ordered the Athenians to choose seven of their finest young men and seven of their finest young women to be sacrificed each year to the bull-man, the Minotaur, as revenge for killing his son.

One year, the group of young men and women included a strong, brave young man called Theseus. Theseus was convinced he had the courage and strength to kill the Minotaur, and he assured the 13 others not to worry. Theseus thought it was high time to put an end to the feeding of his people to the Minotaur – such a waste of young lives!

Now the king also had a beautiful daughter called Ariadne. When Ariadne saw this brave and handsome youth named Theseus she fell in love at first sight. So she decided to help him with his mission because she was afraid he would not succeed, and would end up becoming food for the Minotaur. Ariadne gave him two things to help him on his quest – a sword and a ball of the fleece thread she was spinning.

Her reason for giving the thread was that once Theseus had killed the Minotaur he would be able to find his way out of the maze of tunnels and pathways. Theseus took the sword and the ball of thread, which he fastened to the door when he went in. After killing the Minotaur, he was able to safely make his way out again by gathering up the thread as he followed the maze of pathways.

This is how Theseus saved his own life and the lives of the young men and girls who had been offered to the Minotaur. Emerging from the maze, he sailed with them and Ariadne safely back home.

Craft activity related to the above two stories

After the story, show thin cotton and then show thick thread ...

What if Theseus took a thread into the maze that was so weak it broke? What if you needed a strong thread to take into your cave in the mountain but all you had was a ball of wool? Challenge the group to break a thread of wool (this is easily done). Then discuss twisties (using four to eight threads of wool) that no one can break – see details below!

Twisties

Children to work with a partner. Each pair to take a small ball of wool and stretch it the length of the room, then double it back to make 2 threads the same length (even double it back again to get 4 long threads). Each person in the pair holds an end (2 or 4 threads in their hand) and the threads are stretched out between them. One partner twists one way and the other twists the other way ... the threads are twisted until it is too tight to twist any more; then the twisted thread is doubled back on itself (doubling the strength – 2 threads become 4; 4 threads become 8) and a knot tied at each end to prevent it coming undone.

'Story bones' – The Magic Cloak

Whitehorse, Yukon: two different story ideas written for a child who was very insecure, lacked resilience or any kind of hope, and needed something to pull him 'upwards'. Suitable for age eight and up.

There was once a young boy who was given a special gift when he was born.

This gift was a magic cloak ... magic because it was invisible, and because it held many special powers.

It was woven with threads given by the boy's mother and the boy's father, threads given by all his grandparents and threads given by their parents and grandparents before them. These threads held secrets, secrets of love, secrets of life and secrets of adventure.

All the years the boy was growing up, he loved to wear this magic cloak. In the winter it kept him warm, in the dark night it shone golden to light the way, and in the summer the threads spread wide to allow the cooling breezes in. Because the cloak was invisible nobody knew about it ... it was the boy's best-kept secret.

Soon the boy grew into a strong young man, and as he grew the cloak expanded and grew with him, so it was always a perfect fit. People in his community marvelled at his enthusiasm, his brightness and strength, and were in awe of his special qualities.

Suggested journey (A)

One fine day the young man was hiking in the mountains. A storm came upon him, with winds so strong that his magic cloak was ripped from his back and whirled high into the sky. The youth was helpless in his efforts to stop this, and he watched as his cloak swirled up and across to the rocky mountain cliffs. There he saw it land right at the edge of a cave.

When the storm abated, he climbed up the mountainside and crept close to the bushes near the cave. He could see his coat lying on the sandy floor of the cave, but just behind it a whole family of bears was living. What was the young man to do? He knew he was powerless to face them head on! How was he going to find a way to retrieve his magic coat? [Develop story ...]

Suggested journey (B)

One fine day the young man was hiking in the mountains. A storm came upon him, with winds so strong that his magic cloak was ripped from his back and torn into many pieces. The youth was helpless in his efforts to stop this, and when the storm abated, he collected the parts of his special cloak and carried them back home.

Then began a search for magic threads to stitch his cloak back together ...

How and where was he to find such threads? What would they be made from? How could he gather and use them? [Develop story ...]

14

Sexual Abuse/Sexual Awareness

Yogi and the Cobra Snake
by Edi Grace Ryagard

Note from the author: When I was telling stories in the Knysna community (South Africa) I was made aware that many of the primary school children, particularly in the coloured communities, suffered at the hands of alcoholic and sexually abusive families. The teachers admitted that they could not really become involved by changing their set curriculum on social and cultural guidance, so they were pleased to let me address this theme by telling the story below. It emphasizes that children can find the strength to say no, and will be protected by their teachers and (non-offending) parents. Or at least it suggests that they can seek this care and believe in it.

Of course, the chant throughout and at the end of the story made the children very enthusiastic to shout it all the louder, to sound like they were in charge. I believe that this story gave positive encouragement to some of those children 'affected' by such issues.

There was once a boy called Yogi who lived in a village in a far-off land. Yogi was a happy, healthy child who loved to play; and most of all he loved to play in the forest near his village.

Yogi had a special friend who lived in a cave in the forest – a beautiful cobra snake. Whenever Yogi walked past the cave the cobra would slide out and speak to him, telling him interesting stories and secrets that no one else knew. The cobra's eyes would sparkle and his forked tongue would slip in and out of his mouth in delight. He loved the times when Yogi would stop outside his cave, and one day he even showed Yogi the beautiful hood around his head.

For a long time, Yogi and the cobra stayed secret friends. Yogi was afraid that if he told his parents or friends that he had a cobra snake for a friend, they would laugh at him or they would not believe him.

One day, however, when Yogi stopped on the path to greet the cobra, the cobra invited him into his cave. Yogi was curious to see inside his friend's house and so he followed the cobra through the cave entrance. But once they were inside together Yogi could see how his friend had changed – his eyes were looking wicked, his mouth was hissing and he was standing up high showing off his hood. Then he started to wind his snake body around Yogi and squeezed him until he could hardly breathe, and Yogi was so frightened that he fainted.

When he woke up the snake was there, smiling down at him and talking in soft words: 'You are now my special friend and what happened here today is our special secret. You must never tell anyone – not your parents or teacher or friends – for if you tell our secret I will come to your house and slide under the door and into your bed and my fangs will bite into your neck and you will die. Now go home and tell no one, and promise to return to see me again tomorrow.'

Yogi was very frightened so he made the promise to the cobra; then the cobra allowed him to go home. When he reached his house he went straight to bed and cried and cried. He wanted to tell his mother but was so worried that the snake would come and kill him and his family. And because he had made the promise to return to the cobra's cave he went back there every day after school to play the horrible 'secret' game – he was so scared to do this but he was more scared not to do it as he thought the snake would come and kill his family.

The weeks passed by and Yogi grew sadder and thinner. His teacher and parents became very worried about him. He was no longer the happy healthy child whom they knew from before, but was now sad and sickly looking, and did not want to play with his friends or speak to anyone.

One day after school, Yogi's teacher called him to her and put her arms around him and asked him if he had something he wanted to talk about. Yogi tried to be brave and say nothing, but then he started to cry and said 'He will kill me if I tell, I don't want to die!'

His teacher held him close and said 'Yogi, no one can kill you – you have your parents and teacher to protect you from anyone who threatens you like this. Now tell me who has told you these things?'

But Yogi would not say, and so his teacher explained to him that he had a right to say no to whoever was threatening him and a right to turn around and run away. The teacher helped Yogi learn some strong words to say to protect himself:

Don't you dare, don't you dare, you ugly snake don't you dare touch me,
I will tell, I will tell, I will tell and then I'll be free!

On his way home, Yogi met the cobra on the path and, remembering the words that he had learnt from his teacher, he bravely called out to him:

Don't you dare, don't you dare, you ugly snake don't you dare touch me,
I will tell, I will tell, I will tell and then I'll be free!

Yogi then ran home, and waited for the snake to follow – but, to his surprise, nothing happened. Then his mother and father came into his room and Yogi told them the whole story.

Yogi's parents then gathered many friends with sticks and a bag, and went into the forest to catch the cobra. They found him lying on a rock in the sun and put him in the bag and tied it tight.

Because the cobra was so beautiful he was taken to the zoo in the city and kept in a glass cage for people to look at. The children used to like poking their fingers at him through the glass and saying 'We are not scared of you – you can't bite us.'

Yogi became a healthy, happy boy again who liked to play with his friends – but whenever he went to the forest he was always careful to stay away from the cobra's cave.

And Yogi taught his song to his friends, in case one day they needed to use it:

Don't you dare, don't you dare, you ugly snake don't you dare touch me,
I will tell, I will tell, I will tell and then I'll be free!

The Caterpillar

Written by Marama's group at a workshop at Moruya, NSW. Sometimes, in a therapeutic story-making workshop, an adult needs to process their own childhood traumas through a story. This story is an example of such a situation. It is included in this collection, as the theme of transformation could also be helpful for a child or a teenager.

Note from the author: This is a story-poem written for an adult who was sexually assaulted at the age of three by a stranger in a park. Her brother ran for help and the resulting family distress, which included a visit to the police station for an identity parade, affected her life for many years. This person is now at a mature age, but all her life she has been plagued by a sense of isolation and disconnection. Although she had revisited the issue at an emotional and psychological level (in therapy), writing this story helped her at a more direct, intuitive level to accept the experience without having to understand it. The imagery and the changed point of view brought to the adult woman new layers of meaning and a sense of wonder and transformation.

Caterpillar

On a dark night without any moon,
Caterpillar finds herself changing.
She is being spun
in a cocoon –
deep in a dark cocoon
and she wonders
Will the world ever be the same again?

Round
and round
and round
the spinning wraps her
tight and still –
tight, with no light, until …

the creatures of the forest gather, wonder, worry
How did Caterpillar get in that cocoon?
Why is she there and will she ever be the same again?

Caterpillar whispers,
Don't worry. Give me time.
I'll be out soon
by the light of the moon.
The moon hears Caterpillar's whisper

and sends her starlight fairies
down to help:
pink, green and aqua,
purple, silver, gold,
fairies bring their colours bold –
sparkles spark and sprinkles sprink.
Then, in the blink
of an eye,

one wing unfolds
and then the other
the cocoon splits open

and with a flutter
comes a cry –
the creatures shout
What a surprise!
Our clever and beautiful butterfly!

She fans her wings,
begins to rise,
and all her colours light the sky.

The Princess and the Mirror

This story was written in response to a request from a concerned mother about how to teach 'appropriate ways and places for sexual exploration'. The mother wrote: 'At present my five-year-old daughter is beginning to explore her body in what I believe to be a normal and healthy way. Of course she wants to share her discoveries and delights with her friends. Other families (on our beach-side community) wish to put very firm boundaries in place regarding sex play or even the sharing of emerging ideas around it ... I respect this and I feel we need to understand and respect their boundaries, whilst keeping the door open to my daughter's own explorations in healthy, hygienic and appropriate ways. I feel a story is one of the best and most sensitive ways to express this complex issue to my daughter but am finding it hard to come up with one myself. Can you help?'

After finding out that some of the little girl's favourite interests were dancing and princesses, I wrote 'The Princess and the Mirror', keeping a light and humorous approach to the situation. The mother seemed delighted with it. Here is her response: 'For me this story captures the essence of what we need to impart to her. Absolute freedom for her own experiences with her own body, but a need for privacy and an understanding of what is appropriate or not, with others. Dance away pretty Princess!'

There was once a princess living in a beautiful white castle on the cliffs by the sea.

In the castle were many rooms ... a kitchen with many cupboards full of food, a room with tables and chairs where the princess ate her meals with family and friends, a room with a bath for the princess to wash in, a room with a soft bed for the princess to sleep in, and many more different spaces and places for the princess to play.

The princess's favourite place was a room of mirrors. There was a mirror on every wall, there was even a mirror on the back of the door. Here she loved to look at her beautiful body and dance with herself and stroke her silky skin. Every day she would spend time in the room of mirrors, dancing and playing and playing and dancing.

Life was going along very well until one day, early in the morning, a topsy-turvy wind blew across the land. It blew in through the castle door, and in through the castle windows, and blew in and out of all the rooms.

As the topsy-turvy wind blew around the castle it shifted things out of place: the food was blown out of the kitchen and into the bath-room, the bed was blown out of the bedroom and into the kitchen, and the mirrors were blown off the walls of the room of mirrors and onto the walls of the dining room.

When the wind had blown through the castle and back out to sea, the princess ran from room to room trying to work out how to live in this topsy-turvy place. She tried to have a bath but all the food in the bath made it feel like she was in a pot of soup (and the smell of onions was oh so strong!). She tried to sleep in her bed in the kitchen but the cook was making too much noise chopping the food. She tried to dance and play in front of all her mirrors but she missed the quiet of her own mirror room.

Then early in the morning of the next day something happened. A fresh, rosy-pink wind came in from the sea (*suggest using the child's favourite colour for the wind*). It blew in through the castle doors and in through the castle windows and blew through all the rooms.

As if by magic the rosy-pink wind blew everything back to its rightful place, and the princess was able to continue life as before. She was very happy to have the food back in the kitchen, to have her bath filled with clean sparkling water (and no onions!), and her soft cosy bed back in her bedroom.

But most of all she was happy to have her mirrors back in her special room where she could look at her beautiful body and dance with herself and stroke her silky skin. Every day she loved to spend time in the room of mirrors, dancing and playing and playing and dancing.

'Story bones' – broken dolls, lions and crocodiles

The Broken Doll

A story idea for a 9-year-old girl in the Philippines who had been sexually abused by her grandfather. The girl had regressed in her development. She was happiest when she came back to visit her old kindergarten, playing in the sandpit and making things out of sand.

Story about a doll left lying on the road – its arms and legs smashed by a truck – child finds doll and tries to find someone who could fix it. But no one in her village can do it – everyone said it is too damaged to fix. Eventually an old wise woman says to the child, 'Only you can fix this doll' – and gives the child some magic sand to mould new arms and legs. The child works a long time and shapes new arms and legs, then puts them on her doll; and from then on the girl and the doll become best playmates.

The Calf and the Lion

Nairobi – Médecins sans Frontières: a story idea for a 7-year-old who had been sexually abused, aiming to hep the child find ways to cope with and resolve this.

Story about a mother cow who sleeps in a cowshed each night with her baby calves. One of the calves sleeps near the door of the shed; and each night a lion sneaks close and has a munch on the calf's leg. The calf doesn't want to call out for her mother as she is frightened and doesn't know the right thing to do. Eventually a small animal (an antelope? a hedgehog? – what is most appropriate?) came to the calf's rescue. It had seen what the lion was doing every night; and one night it grew brave enough to make a big noise in the bushes and frighten the lion away.

Crocodile Story

Nairobi: story for a 7-year-old girl who had been imitating mature sexual behaviour at school. (Her mother was a sex-worker – they lived in a little one room shack; the girl would watch the mother at 'work' then see the man leave money. Then the mother would use this money to buy food.) The story was written by 'Felix' – the child's psychologist – in an attempt to help the child 'take back her childhood' – see Chapter One, page 19 for more details of the circumstances and outcome.

Story about a mother bear and little bear (the girl's favourite toy was a stuffed teddy bear) – the bears live in a small house in the forest – mother comes home each day ripped and torn but with some fish to eat – little bear decides to follow mother one day to see where she goes fishing – little bear watches as mother reaches river full of snapping crocodiles, then mother jumps in water to catch fish while the crocodiles are snapping at her.

Little bear wants to help mother, so goes back to river by himself and jumps in water to try and catch fish – then a helping hippo rises out of the water (later the use of 'hippo' was changed to a magic giant rock) and lifts the little bear back onto the bank. Suggests that the little bear go to the forest to look for food – there is honey and fruit in the forest – this is the kind of food that is good for children.

Extension of story: The helping hippo also teaches little bear how to make a canoe to travel on the river and catch fish safely.

15

Shy/Withdrawn/Low Self-esteem

Daisy White

A story for four- to six-year-olds, on the theme of shyness turning into confidence.

It was springtime and the Flower Queen and her helpers had been busy with their pots of bright colours, painting the petal dresses of the springtime flowers.

When all the work was finished, the Flower Queen returned to her flower palace in the garden. Tomorrow was the spring flower ball and the Flower Queen needed her rest.

But one little flower had not been included in the springtime painting. The Flower Queen and her helpers had missed the shy little daisy, still hiding in the bushes in her clean, white petticoat.

Now there was no more colour left to share, so Daisy White didn't have a coloured dress to wear.

Poor Daisy White stayed hiding under the bushes and tucked her head away in shame. What would she wear to the spring flower ball? She knew all her flower friends would be there, in their bright, colourful dresses. But she only had her white petticoat.

Daisy White couldn't sleep that night. She stayed awake, wishing for a coloured dress so bright. Mother Moon looked down from the evening sky and saw Daisy White, wide awake in the night.

Mother Moon called down to her:

Daisy White, Daisy White, why are you awake all night,
Looking so sad in my pale moonlight?

When Daisy White told Mother Moon her story, Mother Moon smiled and said, 'Don't worry little Daisy White, I have a friend who can give you some bright colour.'

Daisy White felt much happier now. How special that Mother Moon was going to ask her friend. Daisy White fell into a deep sleep, wondering who Mother Moon's friend could be.

The next morning, when Daisy White woke up, the golden sun was shining right into the bushes where she was hiding. Daisy White felt warm and different. Daisy White felt something warm and golden and bright and different.

She looked down at herself and saw a beautiful golden heart, right in the centre of a snow-white dress. Daisy White was so happy she almost jumped right off her long daisy stem. Now she was definitely ready to go to the spring flower ball – and everyone at the ball agreed that she was the most beautiful flower of all.

Daisy White never found out the name of Mother Moon's friend, but I think I know who it could have been – do you?

The Shy Robot

Nairobi: a story written for a very shy 8-year-old with a stammer who had difficulty making friends. The boy was fascinated by robot toys.

There was once a robot that lived in a toyshop. When it first arrived it was put on a top shelf all by itself and no one seemed to notice it was there.

The robot had been programmed to talk but was too shy to try out its voice. It just sat there all day long, looking down on everything in the shop. The longer it sat there, the dustier it became. Customers came and went every day – many parents with their children – but no one noticed the robot on the top shelf.

Then one night a robber broke through the door of the shop with a loud crash! He was carrying a large bag and he began to pick up toys from the bottom shelves and put them inside.

Suddenly the robot lit up, spun around several times, and called out:

> *I flash my light and spin around,*
> *I bend down low and touch the ground,*
> *I spin and flash, I make a din,*
> *I spin and flash, I flash and spin.*

The robber got such a fright that he dropped the bag of toys, and ran out through the open window and down the road – never to be seen again!

The next morning when the shopkeeper arrived at the shop he saw the broken door and the bag of toys on the floor. He stood there wondering what could have happened.

Suddenly the robot lit up, spun around several times, and called out:

I flash my light and spin around,
I bend down low and touch the ground,
I spin and flash, I make a din,
I spin and flash, I flash and spin.

The shopkeeper looked up and noticed the robot, and remembered how he had put it up on the top shelf a long time ago and forgotten all about it.

'What are you doing hiding away on the top shelf?' the shopkeeper asked the robot. 'A fine robot like this should be in my window display.'

After the shopkeeper had put all the toys back on their shelves and fixed the broken door, he reached up and took down the robot. He wiped off the dust and put it right in the middle of his toyshop window.

Of course, you can imagine what happened – the robot didn't last very long in the window! A boy came into the shop with his father to choose a birthday present for his ninth birthday. 'That's exactly what I want', he cried out. He reached into the window to pick up the robot and after his father had paid the shopkeeper, they took the robot home.

As soon as the robot arrived at its new home, it excitedly began to spin around and dance and sing:

I flash my light and spin around,
I bend down low and touch the ground,
I spin and flash, I make a din,
I spin and flash, I flash and spin.

The Lonely Robin
by Stephen Sharpe, of Happiness Drum Circles Ltd

A story to encourage participation from the youngest and shyest participants in an out-of-school musical event in northern Scotland.

Webpost from the author: Occasion ... a community out-of-school musical event for 20 × 3–8-year-olds, some of whom know each other and some of whom don't.

Session length = 1 hr.

Drive to the gig = 1 hr.

I'm driving to my music gig and planning the format of the workshop, and I think to myself, wouldn't it be wonderful to start with a story (after only two days of reading Susan Perrow's book!). So I spent the driving time creating a story that might influence the quality of the interaction between the kids, and set the tone for a fun, inclusive, interactive team event ... Well, it was lovely. We all sat round the balafon (xylophone) and I got them joining in with actions and sounds – and they were captivated, and I could see the smaller ones who were clinging on to their mums start to come away and be a part of the main group. After the story I said that we weren't going to build a nest today but some great music instead, and asked them all if they wanted to help us out. They all shouted YES and jumped up with glee. The rest of the session was great as we played games and rumbled, and played more games and rumbled and did some beats, and then a bit more rumbling! – you know how it is! My point is that the story captivated their imaginations, helped the shy ones come away from their mums and join in with the rest of the group, and set the tone for a lovely group experience (whether or not the music was any better quality I doubt very much, but the feeling was there). And I also felt great. I had made up my first ever story!

There was once a robin who was different from all the other robins as he didn't like to play with the other birds. All day long he just sat in his nest eating worms. The other birds would come and call for him from time to time, but he would always decline their invitation and choose to stay in his nest alone.

One day, while he was on the forest floor looking for worms, a great storm blew up and he saw his tree fall, along with his nest. That night was the coldest, loneliest night he ever had. The next day the other birds noticed that his home had gone and they asked him if he wanted help to rebuild it. He accepted their help and slowly, throughout the day, he began to realize that being with the other birds wasn't so bad after all.

In fact, by the end of the day he had made some great friends, and it was only through their combined efforts that the robin had a new home by the time the sun was setting. That night he felt so happy, that he asked his new friends if they would like to stay with him in his nest for the night. They said yes and they had the warmest, cosiest night ever. From that day on the robin never chose to be alone again, he became one of the friendliest birds in the forest, and if ever there was a job to be done to help any of the woodland creatures, he would rally a team of birds together to help out.

The Bunny Clowns

Nairobi: story for a four-year-old boy who was always crying, sad and withdrawn. The parents were very dismal and melancholy about life, and the teachers who worked on this story idea thought that bringing some laughter and fun into the mix could help increase the child's social confidence and skills. I encouraged the teachers to share the story with the parents as well as the child.

There was once a bunny who didn't know how to smile. Mother Bunny tried all she could to make her little bunny smile, but it all seemed a waste of time. Father Bunny tried all he could to make his little bunny smile, but it all seemed a waste of time. Sister Bunny tried all she could to make her little bunny smile, but it all seemed a waste of time.

Then one day Mother Bunny had an idea. She hopped through the forest to visit the wise parrot of the forest and tell him the problem. The wise parrot gave Mother Bunny a basket full of coloured feathers and he sent her back to her bunny hole with a secret plan.

That night, Mother Bunny dressed up in some of the coloured feathers and began to dance. Then Father Bunny dressed up in some of the coloured feathers and began to dance. Then Sister Bunny dressed up in some of the coloured feathers and began to dance.

After watching all this funny dancing, the sad little bunny couldn't help himself – he took some of the coloured feathers from the parrot's basket and he too began to dance.

That night the bunny family had the best time together that they had ever had – they danced and danced until they were so tired they fell into bed and slept all through the night and the next day and the next night.

When they woke up the basket of feathers had mysteriously disappeared, but the sun was shining and they all ran outside and tumbled and played in the sparkling green grass.

Little Polar Bear

A story-rhyme for a three-and-a-half-year-old who is not joining in with group activities. To be done as a finger play/hand-gesture game, or as a simple puppet show with the whole class. The idea came from a workshop in Byron Bay.

Little Polar Bear won't come out today,
He stays in his cave to watch the others play.

Are you there Little Bear? Come out to play.
No, says Little Bear. I'm not ready to play.

Little Polar Bear stays in his cave
The other bears go roly-poly through the day.

Are you there Little Bear? Come out to play.
No, says Little Bear. I'm not ready to play.

Little Polar Bear stays in his cave
The other bears go roly-poly through the day.

Are you there Little Bear? Come out to play.
No, says Little Bear. I'm not ready to play.

Little Polar Bear stays in his cave
The other bears go roly-poly through the day.

Are you there Little Bear? Come out to play.
Yes, says Little Bear. I'm ready to play.

Little Polar Bear leaves his snowy cave
And joins in the roly-poly through the day.

'Story bones' – wizards, fairies, mermaids and mermen

The following story ideas were created at various workshops around the world.

The Wizard's Cloak

Ireland: for a six-year-old child who is withdrawn and not participating.

Child finds a 'wizard's cloak' in grandfather's cupboard – wears it – cloak gives confidence to do certain tasks – list at least three tasks (cloak given to child as a story prop).

Fairy Twinkle

Nairobi: story idea for a very shy three-year-old child

There was once a pink blossom tree full of pink fairies. Each fairy had a home in one of the pink blossom flowers. Down in the grass below a little daisy fairy was hiding. She stayed inside her bud house because she thought she didn't sparkle like the blossom fairies overhead. Then one day a dewdrop landed on her bud house and found its way down inside. The rainbow light in the dewdrop sparkled on the daisy fairy's wings: the bud house opened, and out flew the daisy fairy to meet the world.

The Mermaid who Lost her Voice

New York: story idea for a six-year-old Japanese girl attending an English-speaking school who would not attempt to use English.

Mermaid – born unable to speak – gathering shells one day in a lagoon when a baby bird flies from the forest to the shore and lands in a rockpool nearby – mermaid needs to call the mother bird and needs to call out loud (mermaid can't travel from the water to the forest so needs to call out). She finds her voice, calls the mother and saves the baby.

Merman and Iceberg Story

Stroud: story idea for a very withdrawn eight-year-old child who lacked confidence and self-esteem

Story about a group of mermen – colourfully dressed – living in the rocky caves on the coast – singing together – one merman always on the edge, not wanting to get involved – storm comes and wave washes this merman off the rocks – the currents carry him far out to sea – ends up on iceberg – falls asleep with cold – time passes and then sun shines down and wakes merman with its warmth – merman is so happy to feel the warmth of the sun that he starts to sing – the other mermen hear his song and send a helper (a seal?) to push the iceberg back to the rocky coastline – merman returns to his brothers and they celebrate with much song and feasting.

16

Swearing/Shouting/Silly Speech

The Singing Snake and the Dancing Bear

I wrote this story after a request from a woman in the Philippines who had escaped a difficult domestic abuse situation with her eight-year-old son. She asked for some help for her son's 'foul' language (her words). She wrote 'Though I am a trained art therapist, I feel a bit helpless about how to help my son heal the foul language he picked up from his father as well as the aggressive hostility that comes and goes'. With some clues as to the boy's favourite toys (including 'Bear – the wise one among them all') and his favourite activities (including dancing and music), this snake and bear story emerged.

Email from the mother: Thank you so much for the story that helped my son gently heal his colourful vocabulary. There are still a few 'strays' but they are not so strong now and hardly come out! Because of your story, I have been inspired to create more stories for my son.

There was once a beautiful snake who lived in a large and comfortable basket and travelled with the best circus in the land. As you can imagine, this was not an ordinary snake. Nothing ordinary ever travels with a circus!

This snake was a singing snake! Although he just looked like a plain, black snake, when he opened his mouth he had a long golden tongue, and it was this golden tongue that helped the snake to sing like magic. When the circus arrived in a new town, the snake would be carried in its basket up onto the main stage to perform. He would raise his head high above the edge of the basket and his golden tongue would begin to sing while the audience cheered and clapped.

All across the land the crowds loved the singing snake and this soon became the most popular act in the circus.

However, as years passed by, the snake grew tired of always doing the same thing and always singing the same song, and his performance lost its fresh magic. Sometimes the snake would only feel like singing half a song, sometimes only a few lines, and soon the crowds began to complain that the snake had become lazy.

It then happened that some people began to call out swear-words at the snake on the stage, and the snake, who had never heard such words before, slowly began to repeat these words back to the audience. Some of the members of the audience would roar with laughter, and the snake soon realized that he didn't have to bother singing any more. Instead he could just use a few of these new words to get a response.

But this circus was a family circus, and the ringmaster was not pleased that his singing snake was gaining the reputation of being a swearing snake. The ringmaster didn't know what to do about this, and decided to consult the dancing bear who had been a part of his performing troupe for many years. He knew this bear to be very wise, in fact he had consulted the bear before on many difficult circus matters.

The wise old bear thought for a moment, then said, 'The only way to get our snake to sing beautifully and stop using such foul language is to do this … ' (and the bear bent down and whispered a secret in the ringmaster's ear).

The next day, after the snake had finished his performance, he returned to his basket and fell fast asleep. The ringmaster had been waiting for this moment. Now he could set to work, carrying out the wise bear's suggestions. With many long pieces of grass he wove some thick matting in and out over the top of the basket; and when it was finished, the basket looked as if it were covered with a grass blanket. Inside the basket it was dark and warm, and the snake, thinking it was still night-time, slept a long deep sleep.

Finally the snake woke up and tried to find his way out of the darkness. But when he tried to lift his head out of the basket he bumped against the thick grass blanket. He pushed and pushed, and eventually was able to make a tiny hole in the weaving. He pushed and pushed, and after a long struggle was able to wriggle his way out. The grasses pulled and scratched at his body but slowly and surely he made his way out into the sunshine.

When the snake was out in the sunlight something caught his eye. He turned around and was surprised to see that he had a new, dazzling skin that shimmered with black-and-white diamond patterns.

Squeezing through the tiny hole had pulled off his outer skin. And underneath his plain black skin was this new shining one. The snake began to dance with joy – what a beautiful new skin! The more he danced the more the snake's new skin shimmered and shone, and soon he began to sing as he danced – what a performance that was.

The ringmaster was very happy – his circus now had a dancing singing snake. And the wise bear was very happy – she now had someone to dance with.

Kuky the Kookaburra
by Anatelyah Harari

Note from the author: I wrote this story during your Brisbane writing workshop for a boy (aged five-and-a-half) who used to say 'You're not the boss of me' to people who had advice or 'told' him what or how to do things. The idea for a kookaburra came from watching one bird at dinnertime. When I read it to the children at school there was an audible gasp when Kuky first said those words, 'You're not the boss of me … '. I told it for a week and I must say that I noticed a change in the boy for a while after that. All in all I believe the story had a part in helping him see things from another perspective.

Kuky was a little kookaburra who lived with her family in a gumtree forest amongst beautiful green hills. Many other kookaburra families lived close by, and as Kuky slowly grew she saw her friends grow around her. The kookaburra parents would fly off in search of food for their youngsters, come back with juicy worms and other food and drop it straight into the waiting little mouths.

As time passed some of her older friends started to learn how to fly. They watched their parents carefully and listened to all their instructions and one by one they started taking flight.

Kuky really wanted to fly as well, so she could join her friends, but her mum and dad said she wasn't ready quite yet, she must have patience and wait till the time was right. But Kuky didn't like to wait, she wanted to fly NOW, and since she had been watching her friends learn for a while now, she thought she should be able to do it without any help from anyone.

The next day, when her parents flew off in search of food, Kuky climbed out of her nest and stood on the branch, fluttering her wings. 'You shouldn't try to fly without your parents,' said one of her little friends, 'you aren't ready yet, you're too small.'

Kuky puffed up and said:

You're not the boss of me, I won't listen to you,
Don't tell me who to be and don't tell me what to do!

One of the older kookaburras, who had just returned with some food for her baby, saw Kuky on the branch, getting ready to fly. The older kookaburra said to her: 'You must wait for your lessons in the art of flying, this is how things are done. You are too small and your wings are not ready for flight just yet, so you might hurt yourself if you try.'

Kuky put her wings up to her head and cried out:

You're not the boss of me, I won't listen to you,
Don't tell me who to be and don't tell me what to do!

A little lizard poked its head out of a hole in the tree trunk. 'Kuky, be careful, you aren't ready to fly yet, wait till you grow some more.'

Kuky puffed up and said:

You're not the boss of me, I won't listen to you,
Don't tell me who to be and don't tell me what to do!

Kuky stayed standing on the branch, fluttering her wings. A little wind had picked up and as the breeze blew through the leaves, she thought she could hear it whisper:

Listen and learn
and you will earn
the gift of flight – then like the breeze
you'll fly through the trees.

Just at this moment, her parents came back with some tasty food. They found Kuky still standing on the branch, listening to the song of the breeze.

'Please go back into the nest,' they said, 'it's not time for you to fly yet, you need to grow some more and get stronger. We brought you some juicy worms to help you do just that!'

By this time, Kuky was feeling very hungry and the worms looked delicious. She climbed back into the nest, opened her beak and swallowed her dinner, then snuggled in with the rest of the family. That night she was lulled to sleep by the whispering breeze:

Listen and learn
and you will earn
the gift of flight – then like the breeze
you'll fly through the trees.

Time passed, some days quickly and some days slowly, then one morning Kuky's parents told her, 'You are now strong enough to fly, and we want to teach you just what to do.'

Kuky was so excited. Today was the day for her first lesson in the art of flight.

Kuky listened to everything her parents said and watched everything they did. In no time at all she was flying from tree to tree, catching food and playing with her friends. Like the breeze, she could now fly through the trees! Her heart was filled with joy and she laughed and laughed and laughed.

The Boy and the Pearly White Shell

This story idea came from a group workshop in Wellington, New Zealand. The challenging behaviour concerned a nine-year-old boy who was constantly talking in class. The story resolution is about the importance of listening.

In a coastal village there once lived a young boy who very much wanted a chance to go to sea. He continually asked the fishermen if they would take him out in one of their boats. Every day he would nag and nag and nag at them – 'Take me to sea, take me with you, take me in your boat', he would plead. Finally one of the fishermen agreed, but told the young boy that if he came in his boat he must sit quietly and not talk. 'Talking will scare away the fish!' said the fisherman.

The boat set off and finally reached a good fishing spot; and the fisherman cast his lines. But one minute into the fishing, the young boy began to talk. The fisherman asked him to be quiet but the boy didn't take any notice. The fisherman didn't know what to do – he needed to catch fish to sell at market, but the young boy's constant talking was scaring away all the fish.

Meanwhile dark clouds were gathering overhead. It looked like a storm was on its way, so the fisherman decided to pack up his lines and turn the boat for home.

The young boy saw the storm clouds catching up with the boat and started to call out in fear – but the more he cried out, the quicker and closer the storm clouds seem to be approaching. Finally, the boy was screaming without pause, but there was nothing the fisherman could do. Eventually the storm broke overhead – the rain poured down and the wind blew stronger. Soon large waves were crashing over the boat. One wave caught the boy off balance and he was swept overboard.

Down, down, down he sank – deeper and deeper into the dark blue waters. He sank so deep that he reached the bottom of the ocean; and gleaming on the sand at the bottom was a beautiful pearly white shell. He reached out to pick it up, and the shell, as if by magic, helped to raise him back up to the surface.

By this time the storm had passed, and all was quiet. The fisherman threw out a rope and pulled the boy and his new-found shell out of the water. He wrapped him up in a warm blanket, and headed for home. Soon they were safely back in the harbour.

From this time on, the boy carried his pearly white shell with him wherever he went. He made a velvet bag to keep it in, and every day he would take his shell out of the bag and hold it up to his ear and listen. He could hear the ocean singing a soft song that told how the pearly white shell had saved his life.

A Lyrebird with a Cockatoo Voice

This story idea came from a group workshop in Tasmania – to address a situation with a six-year-old who was constantly talking in a very loud voice. (Note: The lyrebird is an Australian bird that likes to copy other bird sounds.)

When Little Lyrebird was growing up, her best friends were cockatoos.

Squawk, squawk, squawk, squawk, this is how a cockatoo talks.

So squawk, squawk, squawk, squawk, this is how Lyrebird learnt to talk.

One day Little Lyrebird left the part of the forest where the cockatoos were squawking, and she wandered along a path to a place she had never been before.

Something was different in this new place but it took a while for Little Lyrebird to work out what was different. Finally she realized – in this part of the forest there was no squawking. It was so quiet.

It was so quiet that Little Lyrebird could hear the butterflies' wings flapping as they flew across the forest clearing.

It was so quiet that Little Lyrebird could hear the bees buzzing as they flew from flower to flower.

It was so quiet that Little Lyrebird could hear the bellbirds singing from their nests deep inside the bushes.

It was so quiet that Little Lyrebird could hear the kookaburras when they began to laugh high up in the trees.

Little Lyrebird could not believe how many new sounds she could hear. She started to try some different ones – she made a flitter like a butterfly, she buzzed like a bee, she sang like a bellbird, she laughed like a kookaburra.

Little Lyrebird could not believe all the new sounds she was able to make. She was having such fun.

How lucky I am to be a Lyrebird, she thought to herself.

From that day onwards, Little Lyrebird made her nest in this new part of the forest. She still went back to visit her friends the cockatoos, but only every once in a while – she was too busy learning new sounds in her new part of the forest!

The Shouting Clock

This story idea came from a workshop in Singapore and was devised for a three-year-old who always liked to scream. To suit this young age group I suggested the use of a traditional nursery rhyme as a 'story seed':

> *Hickory dickory dock,*
> *The mouse ran up the clock,*
> *The clock struck one, the mouse ran down,*
> *Hickory dickory dock.*

A mouse once lived inside a tall wooden clock. Sometimes the clock would sing to her, *Hickory dickory dock*. When the mouse heard this she would run up the clock and help the clock strike, then run back down again. The mouse was happy to have the clock as a friend and the clock was happy to have the mouse as a friend.

But one day, for no good reason, instead of singing to the mouse, the clock started to shout at the mouse.

HICKORY DICKORY DOCK.

The mouse got such a fright that instead of running up to the top of the clock she ran away to another part of the house and she hid.

The clock didn't know what to do.

The clock missed its friend the mouse, and it missed not having someone to make it strike the way it should.

So the clock shouted even louder:

HICKORY DICKORY DOCK.

But the mouse covered her ears and kept on hiding.

So the clock shouted even louder:

HICKORY DICKORY DOCK.

But the mouse kept on covering her ears, and kept on hiding.

By now the clock had used up all its clock voice, so all it could do was whisper very, very softly:

Hickory dickory dock.

To the clock's great surprise and delight, the mouse came out of her hiding place in the other part of the house, and ran right up to the top of the clock, helped the clock strike, then ran back down again.

From this time onwards, the tall wooden clock always sang or spoke very softly to its friend the mouse.

And the mouse and the clock lived happily together ever after.

'Story bones' – mask men, monkeys, tornados, lions and princes

The following story ideas were created at various workshops around the world.

Mask Man and Houdini

Stroud: story idea for a nine-year-old boy who continually masked his real self by putting on other kinds of silly voices (baby, smart, shouting). The story journey goes from hiding real self to feeling comfortable with true self.

A smart young man who has a lovely home and great car, but then his home is burgled and all is stolen – from then on he withdraws into himself, and turns house into a fortress – then Houdini visits town and breaks in through all his locks (humour here …)

Star Monkey

Nairobi: story idea for ten-year-old who is always using rude language and pushing others away.

A monkey with white patch of fur on chest that looks like a star. This monkey loves to play games with his friends but if they come too close he shouts at them as he doesn't want them to see his star. One day 'star monkey' gets lost and wise tortoise tells him that if he can climb the magic mountain where a special nut tree grows, then one of the nuts from the tree will help him find his way home. Star monkey makes his way up mountain and finds nut (more ideas needed to complete journey …)

The Expanding Tornado

Lismore: story idea for a ten-year-old girl who is always screaming at her mum – who is getting more and more stressed.

Family live on island – quite far from mainland – mum and daughter picking blueberries and see black cloud approaching – daughter starts screaming at mum, cloud grows bigger, daughter screams more, cloud grows even bigger …

The Boy and the Sprinkler

Nairobi: story idea for a five-year-old girl who was adopted soon after birth and has been spitting repeatedly.

An unhappy boy who doesn't like doing all the things that other children like to do when playing out in the playground – he doesn't like jumping on the trampoline, swinging on the swings or running around. But one thing this child does like to do is painting. His teacher has given him some different-coloured clays. He takes the pots of clay and paints pictures all over the side wall of the building. His paintings are so good that everyone in the school comes to admire them.

But one day, the hose is turned on and the sprinkler wets all the paintings on the wall so that they started getting washed off.

The boy is very upset and begins to shout at the hose for doing such damage to his paintings. Then the teacher shows the boy how to turn the hose on and off just enough to get water to mix in with his paints (without the water the clay could dry up). From then on, the hose and the boy became good friends, and together they make many wonderful paintings.

Leo's Roar

Nairobi: story idea for a six-year-old boy who is always shouting at group time.

Migration season – lions are following the herds – one of the lions, called 'Leo' is always roaring at the wrong time and the herds run away. Lions are getting hungry, and also getting very annoyed at Leo. Then a little bird, a wise warning bird, flies down from the trees and lands on a bush next to Leo's head. The bird teaches Leo a song –
  'Roar when you play, not when hunting prey, or you'll scare them away!'

The Cruel Prince

Chengdu: story idea for a ten-year-old child who is always swearing and using 'cruel' words.

Love story – about a handsome but cruel prince who is in love with a beautiful girl – but this girl has a clumsy brother whom the prince does not like. The brother is a builder and one day the prince orders his workers to knock down the house being built by the brother. The brother loses his job and leaves the country. Now the girl refuses to marry the prince. Prince goes to wise man and wise man tells him that to win back his beloved he must get rid of the cruel dragon who lives inside him. To do this he has to rebuild all the houses he has had knocked down – rebuild them with his own hands. Prince works hard and long, rebuilds the house. Girl's brother returns and prince wins back the girl's respect and love.

17

Toileting/Bedwetting

The Barnacle-Covered Fish

At a workshop in Ghilgai, Melbourne, a group worked on a story idea for a six-year-old who kept soiling his pants and was reluctant to sit on the toilet – I have since fleshed out the 'story bones' and created the following story. (Note: the fish metaphor was chosen as the child loves swimming and the sea.) Soiling problems can have deep causes and it's important to remember that a healing story might be part of a whole context of approaches to address the issue.

There was once a school of fish living in a lagoon – they were busy every day swimming, eating and playing.

At the edge of the lagoon was a cave in the reef, and their mother had taught the fish to visit the cave every day to do a rubbing dance against the rock walls. This rubbing dance helped to take off the barnacles that loved to grow on their fishy skin.

One little fish was frightened of the dark cave and would not go in. Day after day went by and he refused to visit the cave. The barnacles kept growing all over his fishy skin and his brothers and sisters started to make fun of him –

Mr Barnacle, looks so funny, all covered over with barnacle bits,
Mr Barnacle, Barnacle Bits.

More days went by and he refused to visit the cave. The barnacles kept growing all over his fishy skin and soon his friends started to make fun of him –

Mr Barnacle, looks so funny, all covered over with barnacle bits,
Mr Barnacle, Barnacle Bits.

Soon the little fish was so covered with barnacles he could hardly swim along. So he found a place to hide amongst the long strands of seaweed. While he was hiding in the seaweed a friendly lobster came swimming by.

'Little Fish, why are you hiding?' asked the lobster.

'I am covered in ugly barnacles and I don't know what to do', said Little Fish.

'Climb on my back', said the lobster, 'I know just what to do'.

And before you could say 'lobster in a pot' the new friend had swum with Little Fish right into the dark cave in the reef. Once inside he helped teach him the rubbing dance and with a rubbing here and a rubbing there, his fishy skin was soon all clean and shining again.

'Thank-you Lobster, I feel so so good,' said the Little Fish.

As he was leaving the cave he looked around. He was surprised that he could see many other little fish, just his size, inside the cave. They were all doing a rubbing dance, rubbing off barnacles against the rock walls of the cave, and then swimming back outside.

In fact the cave was not as dark inside as it had looked from outside!

In fact the little fish could see quite well!

He waved goodbye to the lobster and swam back outside the cave to play with his brothers and sisters and all his friends. Now that all the barnacles had been rubbed off, the little fish could swim faster than ever before. What fun he was able to have, darting here and darting there. He was so happy that he had learnt a way to rub off all the barnacles from his fishy skin.

The Gum Tree
by Natalie

Note from the author: Here is my story of 'letting go', written for my little boy who became afraid to let go of his poos just before he turned three (something that had previously always been so effortless for him). He would do all he could to stop doing a poo – standing on his head, spending a lot of time upside down, running around – never able to sit still or indeed focus on any other aspect of life. He was so anxious and would call out to me 'Mummy mummy mummy, help me' every few minutes; and every time he had an urge to go he would scream and cry. This could go on all day every day until a poo came – one time he even held on for nine days! This went on for eight months and nothing I could say or do ever helped him.

As luck would have it, I was able to attend one of your workshops. Wanting to help my little boy lighten his anxiety around his poos, by the end of the workshop I had come up with this story about letting go. That evening I told him the story as he was going to sleep. He became very still and fully engaged by it and asked for it every night thereafter. I continued to tell this story over the next few nights; and on the fourth day, he quietly took himself off behind the curtain and did his poo (in his nappy) with no fuss or anxiety – and just said afterward 'Mummy I did my poo'. Delighted by this breakthrough and progress, I continued with this story nightly, and every day he would either take himself off into the dark of the cupboard or behind the curtain and happily do his poos calmly in his nappy. I'm happy to report that seven months down the track (at age 4 years, 3 months) he is out of nappies and pooing in the loo. My little boy has a fabulous imagination, loves being in nature and adores babies so I came up with this story about 'The Gum Tree'. After the success of this story, I find that I am using his toys (e.g. a wooden tree-house and some gum-nut babies) to act out any story or behaviour for him. These stories and rhymes have had profound, far-reaching effects, and have proved much more effective than any other kind of talking or reassuring. It's been like magic watching him work out his fears or concerns through a simple, prop-supported story. This whole process has been a joy and an invaluable tool, and brought some much-needed peace into our household.

In the middle of a beautiful rainforest stood a tall gum tree. This special tree was a home for lots of animals – the laughing kooka-burras, snoozy koalas, playful possums, leaping lizards, friendly frogs, chattering cockatoos, colourful rosellas and rainbow lori-keets – all singing their pretty songs. The gum tree loved to have so many animal friends come to visit and play each day. But the gum tree's most special friends were two gum-nut babies. They wore little gum-nut hats, gum-leaf trousers, gum-leaf shirts and green gum-leaf boots. The gum-nut babies would sing as they danced up and down the gum tree, polishing all the branches with smooth eucalyptus-smelling gum leaves until the gum tree's branches all gleamed and glinted in the sparkling sunshine.

The gum tree was so happy watching all his friends play in his branches. But one day it grew very windy. The wind blew stronger and stronger and as the wind blew, it tugged and tugged at all the gum tree's leaves. The gum tree didn't want to let go of his leaves. The leaves were his friends. They kept him company, kept him warm at night. He couldn't let them go – what would the koalas eat? So he held on tight to them. But the wind blew and blew and blew and shook the leaves and soon one by one the leaves tumbled down to the bottom of the tree. The gum tree was so sad.

But then the gum tree noticed something. He could hear the gum-nut babies singing a little song, 'Leaves, leaves blow away, come again another day.' They sang the song as they busily collected all the leaves that floated down to the ground. 'Leaves, leaves blow away, come again another day.' They sang this song as they swept the leaves into little piles. 'Leaves, leaves blow away, come again another day.' They sang as they gathered the leaves into their little brown sacks on their backs. They were very happy.

The gum tree watched them giving handfuls of leaves to the kangaroo who lived in the shade of the gum tree below. They gave leaves to the ants on the ground to build a home. They gave leaves to the beetles to sleep in. They took leaves to a platypus who lived in a nearby stream, and the gum tree could see snuffly wombat snuffling through his lovely bed of soft leaves. All the animals were so happy to have the gum tree's leaves.

The next morning when the sun came up, the gum tree noticed fresh new green leaves bursting out on all his branches. The wriggly caterpillars were happily creeping and crawling on these juicy leaves and the snoozy koalas were licking and smelling and munching these delicious new leaves.

So from that day onwards, whenever the strong wind blew, the gum tree happily let go of his leaves, knowing that new leaves would come again another day.

The Leaking Roof

A story for bedwetting ... for age five and up. This is a light-hearted approach to the problem, that might also need addressing in other ways too, to find the deeper cause or insecurity.

There was once a bed that lived in a child's bedroom in an old wooden house.

This bed loved to do what a bed likes to do best – it loved to help a little child snuggle up cosy and sleep all night. It especially loved to be warm and dry, so it could keep the little child warm and dry all night.

But late one afternoon a storm passed overhead, with clouds heavy with rain. The rain started to fall on the roof of the house – pitter-patter, pitter-patter – and it rained and it rained and it rained. It rained all through the night and all the next day and all through the next night.

The roof of the old wooden house began to leak – drip drip drip. It began to leak so much that water slowly began to fall – drip drip drip – down onto the warm, dry bed.

The roof was so upset. 'My work is to protect my house,' it cried out. 'How can I do good work and keep my house dry if I have holes in my skin?'

There was a wise owl living in the gum tree next to the house. He heard the roof crying out for help. Being so wise, the owl knew just what to do. He quickly collected some gum nuts in his beak and flew down and plugged up all the holes in the roof.

After this help from the wise owl, the roof stopped leaking. No more drip drip drip down onto the little child's bed. From that time on, the bed stayed warm and dry and the little child slept all night long, dreaming sweet dreams about birds and bees and butterflies and trees (and owls and gum-nuts too!).

Good Night, Sleep Well and Bless You

A story for bedwetting rewritten by Susan Perrow from a traditional African tale narrated by Joan Atieno at a storytelling training workshop. Suitable for age five and up.

Once upon a time there was a good woman who lived in a market village near a river. She lived alone in a mud hut with a roof of grass and a wonderful garden where she grew all kinds of fruits and vegetables.

This woman loved children very much but didn't have any of her own. Every night she walked along the dusty paths, visiting all the other huts in the village. She would take fruits from her garden to the children and tell them stories, then she would say 'Good Night, Sleep Well and Bless You.'

One night, as the good woman was travelling along the path to deliver her fruits and say goodnight to all the village children, she met an old woman she had never seen before. The old woman, who was dressed all in white, said, 'I know you and I know what your wishes are, and I am here to grant them. When you reach your hut tonight you will find three little children waiting for you – name them "Good Night", "Sleep Well" and "Bless You".'

'Thank-you, thank-you', said the good woman, as the mysterious old woman in white disappeared along the path towards the river. She excitedly continued her rounds of all the huts, giving out fruits and saying 'Good Night, Sleep Well and Bless You' to all the children, then she hurried home.

When she came closer to her hut, she saw that a light was shining from a lamp that she had not turned on herself. She ran forwards and opened the door, and there, on three new little beds, sat three little children. They ran and embraced her happily. The woman named the youngest one 'Good Night', the middle one 'Sleep Well' and the eldest one 'Bless You'. She went into her kitchen to make some food and she found three little bowls, three little spoons and three little cups, all waiting on the table.

After they had eaten together as a family, the woman tucked her new children into their beds, told them some stories, and said 'Good Night, Sleep Well and Bless You'.

Early the following morning, the three children woke up and found that they all had wet beds. Worried that this might annoy their new mother, they took their bedding down to the river for washing. While they were busy at the river, an old woman, all dressed in white, came to meet them and promised help with their bedwetting. She told them they had to catch three white rabbits and bring them back to her. After hanging out their bedding to dry, the children set out to the forest to look for rabbits. But the rabbits ran too fast for them and the children were not able to catch any. They returned to the old woman down by the river and she sent them home with their dry bedding, saying, 'I will give you an easier task – you each need to find a white feather and then keep it under your pillow.'

The three children returned home, remade their bedding, then helped their mother prepare the food for dinner. After they had eaten together as a family, the woman tucked her new children into their beds, told them some stories, and said 'Good Night, Sleep Well and Bless You'.

At midnight that night, the three children were woken up by a 'knock-knock-knock' outside the window. When they looked out they saw a beautiful white bird sitting in the tree and under the tree, lying on the grass, were three white feathers. They crept outside and collected the feathers and hid one under each of their pillows. Then they went back to sleep. In the morning when they woke up they were amazed to discover that their beds were dry. Straight away the children went to wake up their mother and tell her the whole story. Their mother hugged them all and told them that she knew this old woman to be a very wise helper. She then told them to each keep their magic white feather under their pillows.

The mother and her three children, 'Good Night', 'Sleep Well' and 'Bless You', never saw the old wise woman again. But each of the children kept their magic white feather under their pillow and never again did they find wet beds in the morning.

A Doll called 'Rainbow'

Brightlight was orphaned at the age of six when both her parents died of Aids – she has now been sponsored to attend the Mbagathi Steiner School (organized by African Leaf) in Nairobi where she will live until the age of 15 or 16. Brightlight's story was told to her by her boarding mother. At the same time she was given a special doll dressed in clothes of all colours of the rainbow. Bright took it straight to her bed and tucked it in, under the blanket – so she'd be able to cuddle it to sleep that night. Bright had been wetting the bed consistently since her parents had died. From the night she heard the story and cuddled the doll to sleep, the bedwetting slowly stopped.

Bright Light's mother and father were safe in heaven. Their daughter, Little Bright, was still living down on earth.

At night in the light of the twinkling stars, Bright's parents could see their little daughter asleep in her bed. They were so happy that she had a safe new home and a new mother to take care of her. But they could see that their daughter was sad and lonely sometimes and they wanted to send down a gift from heaven – the gift of a little friend for Bright to play with and to sleep with at night.

With the help of heaven's angels they gathered coloured threads from the rainbow, and on the heavenly weaving loom they wove a special cloth to use to make a little doll.

When the doll was ready, one of heaven's angels cradled her in her arms and travelled with her across the sky of twinkling stars and down to earth. When she arrived at Bright's new house she gave the doll to the boarding mother to give to Bright.

Bright tucked the doll into her bed to sleep with her that night, keeping her warm and cosy. She was so happy to have this gift to play with and sleep with. She named her 'Rainbow', and the doll became her special friend.

'Story bones' – dandelions, house of 'poos' and sea gardens

The following story ideas were created at various workshops.

The Dandelion in the Rain

Chengdu: story idea for a four-year-old boy who wets the bed and also wets his pants during the day.

Story about a dandelion growing next to a river at the foot of a mountain. Butterfly is its friend. One day some rain falls from the clouds and dandelion gets wet. The dandelion asks the butterfly – Can you help me? – I don't like being cold and wet – so butterfly flaps its wings to make dandelion dry. The dandelion keeps growing. Then the rain falls again, this time stronger. The dandelion gets soaking wet and calls out for help. Sun comes to rescue – hears the dandelion calling out so shines down to make it dry. Time passes and soon dandelion gets its first flower – rain comes again. The dandelion calls out – I don't like being wet and cold – help! This time the wind comes and blows the dandelion seeds to many safe places, and many little dandelions start to grow.

The House of Poos

Chengdu: story idea for a six-year-old boy who doesn't want to 'let go' of his poos

Story is about two poos that live in the same house, one called 'Popo' and one called 'Nnn' – Popo is very social and likes to go out – but Nnn likes to stay home alone.

One day Popo leaves home for good, and new friends come to live in the house. Nnn misses Popo – house is now crowded with all the new friends – finally Nnn gets brave enough to leave home and go out into the world.

The Sea Garden Playground

Taruna: story idea for three-and-a-half-year-old boy who was pooing in the kindergarten garden and not using the toilet.

Story about a beautiful underwater garden – with many patterned fish – all playing together in a coral and seaweed garden. But one day a visiting fish comes along and makes a fishy mess all over the coral – the other fish don't know what to do so they try to chase away the visitor as they don't want fishy mess all over their playground – but the visitor keeps coming back as it really wants to play – so the other fish ask wise turtle – wise turtle shows them a hole in the rocks, a deep cave, a place for fishy mess – visitor starts to use this hole for its fishy mess and all is well once again in the underwater garden.

18

Obstinacy/Lack of Social Sense

Little Siafu and her Shiny Stone Drum

The story of an uncooperative safari ant who didn't want to stay in line …

Note: Although children need to grow into independence and freedom, there are times when it is important and/or helpful to be part of a group – e.g. rest time at kindergarten, mealtimes at home and at school, school outings, swimming in deep water, just to name a few! This story is a light-hearted attempt to capture the mood of belonging to a group – it could be used with age three and upwards, and even with primary ages, as a starting point for discussion of group expectations. 'Siafu' is the Kiswahili word in East Africa for safari ant – these ants are seen marching in long lines, one by one, across the plains or through the bush after the rains.

Once again the safari ants were on the move! The short rains had started, and their ant home was no longer warm and dry – in fact it was fast filling up with water. The safari ants were now in search of higher and drier ground.

Little Siafu was at the end of all the ants, struggling to keep up. Ahead of her, the others were stretched out, marching one by one. The line seemed to go on for ever and ever! 'Come on', called her friends, 'or you will be left behind.'

To help her keep step, they started to sing:

The ants go marching one by one, hurrah! hurrah!
The ants go marching one by one, hurrah! hurrah!
The ants go marching one by one, the little one stopped to play on her drum,

And they all went marching, up and around, to get out of the rain,
boom, boom, boom.

Little Siafu was trying to keep step with the song, but it seemed
such a boring thing to do! Finally she decided she didn't want to stay
in line any longer. 'I don't want to stay in line one more minute', she
said to herself. 'I just want to stop, and sit, and play on a drum – just
like the little ant in the song!'

Little Siafu sat down and started to beat time on one of the shining
stones at the edge of the track. As she played she sang a different song
from the one her friends were singing:

I'm tired of having to walk in line, I'm sick of having to keep in time,
I just want to sit in the sun, sit in the sun and play on my drum!

And as she sang and played, the ants kept marching on ahead of
her, one by one, until they disappeared over the hills and out of sight.

Now Little Siafu was all alone.

But not for long!

A brown cricket flew into a bush nearby. 'Play and dance with me',
called out Little Siafu, and the cricket started to make music through
the leaves in the bush. But it was far too LOUD!

Little Siafu cried out:

Please go away and leave me be,
You are far too LOUD to play music with me.

Once again Little Siafu was all alone. But not for long!

A tortoise came plodding through the grass by the track. 'Play and
dance with me', called out Little Siafu, and the tortoise lifted his head
and started to slowly sway from side to side. But it was far too SLOW!

Little Siafu cried out:

Please go away and leave me be,
You are far too SLOW to play music with me

Once again Little Siafu was all alone. But not for long!

A golden weaver bird landed on a tree nearby. 'Play and dance
with me', called out Little Siafu, and the weaver bird started to flit
and dance from branch to branch. But it was far too FAST!

Little Siafu cried out:

Please go away and leave me be,
You are far too FAST to play music with me

Once again Little Siafu was all alone. But not for long!

An elephant came tramping down the track. 'Play and dance with me', called out Little Siafu, and the elephant started to tramp and dance and make music. But the elephant was far too BIG!

In fact Little Siafu was very lucky she didn't get trampled on. She cried out:

Please go away and leave me be,
You are far too BIG to play music with me

Once again Little Siafu was all alone, sitting by the track and playing on her drum. The more she played, the more she realized how much she missed her ant friends.

Soon she found herself singing a different tune:

I wish my friends and I could walk in line,
I wish my friends and I could keep in time,
I don't want to sit in the sun,
I want to walk with my friends and play on my drum!

Suddenly she stood up and picked up her shiny stone drum and started to walk along the path, playing as she went. Faster and faster she walked, along the path, and over the hill …

And over another hill …
And over another hill …
And over another hill …

UNTIL

THERE WERE HER FRIENDS, WALKING IN LINE,
THERE WERE HER FRIENDS KEEPING IN TIME!

Little Siafu was so happy! She caught up with her friends, and proudly walked at the end of the long ant line, playing her shiny stone drum. It no longer seemed boring as she went along!

And as she played her drum she taught her friends a new ant song:

The ants go marching one by one, hurrah! hurrah!
The ants go marching one by one, hurrah! hurrah!
The ants go marching one by one, the little one playing her shiny stone drum,
And they all went marching, up and around, to get out of the rain, boom, boom, boom.

The Digger that Always Says No!

This story idea came from a workshop in Sydney – the group wanted a creative approach for an uncooperative four-year-old who said 'No' to everything. They came up with this story idea and a little rhyme – 'The digger says no, so nothing can grow!' When I heard that my grandson was going through a 'No' stage, I took these story bones and added 'flesh' to finish the story.

There was once a strawberry farmer who owned large fields of strawberries. Every year in the springtime the farmer needed to dig many holes in her fields to plant more strawberry runners. But there came a time when there were too many holes for her to dig by hand, so she decided to go to town and buy herself a digger machine. The digger was linked up to the back of the farmer's car and she slowly towed it all the way home.

'This new digger will save me so much work', said the farmer as she proudly showed her two children. The digger was given a special garage to live in, its fuel tank was filled to the top, and the children helped to scrub and rub it down till it shone bright red. That night the farmer went to bed feeling very happy that she had a new helper on her farm.

The next morning, when the farmer woke up, she went to the garage and climbed into the seat on top of the digger, ready to begin work. She turned the key to the engine, but to her surprise, instead of the engine starting up, a voice called out:

The digger says no, so nothing can grow!

The farmer was so surprised that she almost fell out of her seat. A digger that could talk! She turned the engine key again, and once more a voice called out:

The digger says no, so nothing can grow!

By now the farmer was feeling cross. She had work to do! She spoke loudly to the digger ,'How am I going to dig holes for my strawberry runners if my new machine won't work?' But once more a voice called out:

The digger says no, so nothing can grow!

This time the farmer climbed down from the digger and walked around it, banging it here and banging it there. She was feeling very very cross! 'I'll get you started somehow' she cried out.

But once more a voice called out:

The digger says no, so nothing can grow!

Now the farmer didn't know what else to do, so she decided to go into her house and make a cup of tea. This would give her time to think, and drinking a cup of tea usually helped her find an answer.

While the farmer was busy boiling the kettle to make her tea, her children were busy playing outside in their sandpit. The boy was digging deep holes in the sand with his plastic spade, and the girl was filling the holes with buckets of water. They were having such fun!

But all of a sudden the boy's plastic spade hit the rocky bottom of the sandpit and snapped in half. 'Oh no' cried the boy, 'how am I going to dig holes in the sand with a broken spade?'

'Oh no' cried the girl, 'how will I be able to make pools of water if my brother's spade is broken?'

All this time, the new digger had been looking out of his garage and watching the children playing in the sand. When the spade snapped in half, the digger came to life. Its lights flashed, its engine whirred and purred, and all by itself it drove out of the garage. It pulled up by the sandpit and with one large movement it had dug the deepest hole the children had ever seen.

The children laughed and the digger laughed, and the children used buckets and filled the hole with water. The digger dug some more holes, and they all laughed some more. When the farmer finished her cup of tea and came outside the house, she saw what had happened, and she also laughed. Her new digger now knew how to be a digger!

The farmer climbed up onto the machine and set off to her fields. Together they worked through the day till all the holes had been dug for the strawberry runners. The children helped to plant the straw-berries, and when all the work was done, the digger helped dig more holes in the children's sandpit. In return the children helped keep the digger clean and shining bright. It sat in its garage each night feeling very proud that it now knew how to be a digger.

Soon there were ripe red strawberries for the farmer to take to market, and plenty of strawberries for the children to eat for breakfast each morning. The farmer was happy, the children were happy, and the digger was happy!

A Friend on the Farm
by Edna Sophi Amunga

A lovely story with a strong sense of community about how friends and helpers often come to us in unexpected and unplanned ways. It can be told with a simple prop made from two crossed sticks tied together with a simple dress over the top. An upside-down bell-shaped flower could be used to make the hat (this is how the writer shared the story at the teacher-training course in Nairobi). The songs can be sung in Kiswahili or English. Suitable for four years and up …

There once lived a farmer who had a wife who was a washerwoman. Every morning, the farmer would wake up and go to his fields to dig and plant and harvest, but he had to spend most of his time chasing away crows that were eating his maize. His wife would go from house to house collecting clothes to wash. She would wash them and hang them up to dry then return them in the evening all clean, dry and folded.

Everyday, as the farmer was chasing the crows, tsa, tsa, he would sing:

Kunguru wanakula mahindi shambani; Nani atanisaidia kuwafukuza?
(The crows are eating maize in the farm; who will help me chase them away?)

This crow chasing went on for days and days, until one day the farmer fell ill. His wife had to take care of him as well as get her washing work done. She didn't have any spare time to go to the fields and chase the crows. The farmer was worried about his maize but there was nothing he could do but lie in bed and sing:

Kunguru wanakula mahindi shambani, Nani atanisaidia kuwafukuza?

One day, the farmer's wife woke early, washed her dress and some of the farmer's shirts and trousers, then hung them on the line. Then she set off to collect clothes from her neighbours so that she could do her washing work. In the late afternoon she removed the dry clothes but forgot to take down her dress from the end of the hanging line.

That night there was a strong wind. It blew from side to side, and the dress was blown from side to side. As the wind got stronger, tap! went off one peg from the dress; and tap! went off the other peg. The dress was blown up in the sky and across the farm and then landed upon a small dead tree that had been growing in the middle of the maize fields.

The next day the farmer woke up feeling better and he decided to go to check on his maize. When he reached close to the fields he saw someone standing in the middle of the maize. 'That must be a thief' he thought, and slowly he crept closer and closer. As he was getting closer, the wind started to blow and the 'thief' started to move a little. Then the farmer saw that it was not a thief but it was his wife's dress hanging on an old dry tree.

The farmer was very surprised! 'This is a new friend sent to guard my farm from all the crows' he thought. He was so happy that he ran to his wife and told her about their new friend. Together they found an old hat and set off to place it on the new friend's head. They called the friend 'scarecrow' and from that day onwards it helped to scare away all the crows, leaving the farmer more time to do his farming work.

Kunguru wameenda, enda, enda; kunguru wameenda juu angani.
(The crows have gone, gone, gone; the crows have gone up to the sky)

Twiga in the Mist

A story for children aged five to eight about cooperation and helping, based on nature observations in Kenya. Note: Twiga is the Kiswahili word for giraffe, and Simba is the Kiswahili word for lion.

Lady Mist is swirling, swirling, filling the valleys all around,
Lady Mist is thick and curling, covering the earth without a sound.

It was early in the morning, and Mother Giraffe was taking her new baby down to the river for his first drink. She was walking very slowly so that her little one, with his very short giraffe legs, would be able to keep up with his mother with her very long giraffe legs.

But as they crossed over the hill and started down the rocky path into the valley, without any warning Lady Mist swirled up to meet them. Swiftly and silently she curled her thick white dress around baby giraffe and within a few minutes he was separated from his mother and wandering all alone. His mother's tall head was stretching up and out of the swirling whiteness, but little giraffe was hidden deep inside.

Mother Giraffe was very worried! She bent her long neck down to look for her baby, but she couldn't see anything in the thick white mist.

And then she heard a sound that filled her with fear. It was the growling of Simba, first ever so faint, and then growing louder and louder. Simba the lion was also on his way to the river this morning!

Simba is coming, over the hill he comes,
Great Simba comes now – Twiga beware! Twiga beware!

Mother Giraffe frantically looked around for help. Then she saw her friends, Dudu the dove and Didudidu his wife, sitting together on the branch of an acacia tree that was also stretching up out of the swirling mist.

'Please, Dudu and Didudidu, fly out to find our brother the wind, and ask him to come and blow away Lady Mist. Please hurry, so I may find my baby before Great Simba comes down the path and has him for breakfast.'

The doves listened and soon they too heard the growling of Great Simba coming down the path.

Simba is coming, over the hill he comes,
Great Simba comes now – Twiga beware! Twiga beware!

The doves of course wanted to help their friend Twiga, so they flew up and across the plains looking for Brother Wind. They hadn't gone far when they found Brother Wind playing round and round in circles with the red dust on the plains. He was delighting in teasing a herd of zebra by changing their white stripes into red ones. Dudu called out:

'Please Brother Wind, come and blow away Lady Mist from the valley. Please hurry, so Mother Giraffe can find her baby before Great Simba comes down the path and has him for breakfast.'

When Brother Wind heard that Mother Giraffe needed help, he stopped playing his teasing game with the zebras, and quickly followed Dudu across the plains and down into the valley.

*

Meanwhile, back in the valley, Great Simba had almost reached the place where Mother Giraffe was waiting. The thick white mist was still swirling around her long legs and hiding her baby – somewhere, somewhere!

> *Simba is coming, over the hill he comes,*
> *Great Simba comes now – Twiga beware! Twiga beware!*

Simba walked carefully around Mother Giraffe – he knew not to risk going anywhere near her long 'kali' legs. Then through the mist he kept walking, following the path and following a very sweet baby nyama (meat) smell, which seemed to be growing sweeter and stronger with every step he took.

Then, just in time, Dudu and Didudidu flew down into the valley, with Brother Wind following close behind. They had come past the mountain where Sister Rain had been resting, and the wind was blowing some of her clouds in front of him.

When they reached the valley, the wind and the rain joined together, firstly with a slow ha-whooo, ha-whooo, ha-whooo, and a gentle pitter-pat, pitter-pat, pitter-pat, and then building up to a loud storm (make storm sound with fingers and hands).

Then, all was quiet!

As quickly as Lady Mist had arrived, the storm had washed it away. Great Simba, who didn't like getting his paws wet, turned to follow the path out of the valley and back to the dryness of the wide-open plains.

And when Mother Giraffe looked around for her baby, she found him just close by, huddled under a large acacia tree – the very same tree where her friends, the doves, lived.

She bent down and licked all over his face and body with her long tongue (which is how a giraffe mother hugs and kisses her baby!)

And Dudu and Didudidu sat on the top branch of their acacia tree, resting after their long journey, and watching and smiling quietly to themselves.

When Mother Giraffe lifted her head again she saw that Sister Rain had filled a large pool in the rocks at the top of the valley. The water sparkled in the sunshine and seemed to be calling 'Come and drink me, Come and drink me'. So mother and baby walked to the rock pool and had a long drink together.

And, from that day onwards, until her baby had grown tall like her, Mother Giraffe always looked for pools of drinking water in the rocks at the top of the valley, left by the rain after the storms. She was careful never again to go down to the river early in the morning, in case Lady Mist was waiting in surprise to hide giraffe babies in her white swirling dress.

> *Lady Mist is swirling, swirling, filling the valleys all around,*
> *Lady Mist is thick and curling, covering the Earth without a sound.*

The Keeper of the Lake

A story for Taylor's Lake, Byron Bay (a sacred aboriginal site) – written to help encourage community involvement in the protection of the fore-shores of the local lake from development. The story was told to about a hundred children and parents on the sand at the edge of the lake, and then everyone helped build a symbolic sand wall across the entrance. This creative strategy attracted media attention, and front page photos of children building the protective wall were published in several papers. The development never went ahead!

The Keeper of the Lake looked in her magic mirror, the one that always told her what was happening in the world around her home. But today, instead of seeing the golden sun shining, the birds happily building their nests, or the rainbow after the rain, she could only see dark storm clouds filling the sky.

She sighed a great sigh – straight away she knew that this was not an ordinary storm approaching. These were the storm clouds of war, the start of a great battle that she had been warned about for a long time. Already the roar of engines and the high-pitched sounds of machines could be heard on the edge of the forest surrounding her lake.

She called together the wise spirits of the bush to prepare them for the difficult times ahead. 'Our only chance' she said 'is to form a mighty ring through the forest around the edge of the lake, like a great castle wall, woven through and through with bush-land magic and strong enough to stop any kind of force breaking it down. Go and gather as many animals and birds as you can, and ask them to spread out, side by side, to make this great circle together.'

And so the wise bush spirits took the message to the bush-land animals and birds and slowly a wall through the forest started to take shape around the lake, stretching from the south to the west and the north. On the ground, the lizards, snakes and frogs and many other animals gathered side by side, while above them in the bushes and trees the birds stretched wing-tip to wing-tip. Even the pelicans came to lend their great wings to build this special wall.

Then the bush spirits wove their bush magic through and through the wall, with the giant banksia men making it strong and the wattle fairies filling all the gaps with their golden light.

But at the lake's entrance on the ocean side, where there was no bush-land at all, the circle was not complete. 'Who can help here?' the Keeper of the Lake asked her magic mirror.

Then she saw the children coming down to the beach to see what they could do. With eager hands and much chatter and laughter they built a wall of sand and sticks and flowers and shells, right across the entrance to the lake, completing the magic ring.

The Keeper of the Lake looked in her magic mirror and saw that the circle wall was now complete, doing its good work in guarding her sacred waters. She smiled to herself, content and happy, knowing that this magic ring would protect the lake, once and for all, from any kind of danger.

A Gift of Shells

A story for five- to seven-year-olds to encourage cooperation and a sense of helping/sharing.

There once lived a very old gnome in a cave in the rocky cliffs by the sea. With the rest of his gnome family he spent all his time knocking and scraping and tapping and digging for crystal treasures in the rock walls of his home. He had worked so hard for so long that his old back was bent and sore, and his arms and legs had lost much of their strength.

One day this old gnome decided to say good-bye to the younger members of his gnome family and set out to look for a new home for himself. He knew that it was time for him to leave – he wasn't much help anymore and he only seemed to be getting in the way. And so began a long, slow journey for him along the rocky seashore. He travelled until he came to a golden stretch of beach where many sand hills sloped down to the water's edge. With his old and tired arms he found he could dig quite easily into the soft side of one of these hills, and he set to work digging a new cave home, a sand-cave home. He collected driftwood to strengthen its walls and make his table, and used seaweed for his bed. When his digging and building work was finished he ate a filling meal of sea-foam pancakes and then lay down for a long sleep on his soft seaweed bed.

Time passed, and the old gnome settled quite happily into his new sand-cave home. He missed his gnome family back in the rocky cliff cave, but he soon made new friends on the seashore with the different beach creatures and sea birds that lived there. They were glad to have this little gnome now living with them, and because his beard and hat and clothes always seemed to be full of sand, they called him Sandy, Sandy the beach-gnome.

Sandy was kind and good to everyone, and he kept himself busy caring for any new friends in need. He nursed the lost baby seagulls; he rescued little fish stranded in the shallow rock pools; he carried the orange star-fish that had been washed high up on the beach back down into the water; he gathered piles of sea-foam to make pancakes – and each day he shared these with the little crabs who sought the protection of his sand-cave home when high tide washed its waves far up the beach.

However, even though he had made many new friends and found new tasks to keep him busy, there was one thing from his old cliff cave home that Sandy still missed very much. He remembered the beautiful crystal treasures that used to shine like stars in the night sky in the walls of the rocky cave, and often he would sigh to himself 'Oh how I wish I had beautiful treasures like that in my new sand-cave home. The seaweed and driftwood seem very drab and dull compared to the sparkling crystals in the walls of my old home.'

Now the little crabs heard Sandy make this wish one day, and they decided they would try to help it come true. They told it to the silver fish who then swam far out in the sea to the great rock castle of their Sea Queen, the queen of the mermaids.

Basking on a warm rock she lay, her rainbow tail glinting in the sunlight, and her mermaids-in-waiting swimming in the clear blue waters all around her. The silver fish whispered Sandy's wish to the Sea Queen, who had already heard stories of this good little beach gnome who was so kind to all her sea creatures that lived along the shore. She smiled down at the silver fish and said she would like to give Sandy a gift, a gift from her sea kingdom, a gift that would make his wish come true.

Calling her mermaids to the edge of her rock castle she threw down a great netted bag to them. 'Take this to the far reaches of my sea kingdom and gather up as many beautiful shells as you can find. Return with it only when the bag is filled to overflowing with my glistening sea treasures.' The mermaids then took hold of the great netted bag and set off swimming into the deep waters below. For many days and many nights they swam, searching the sea floor for shells of all patterns and sizes and shapes, and slowly filling the bag with beautiful sea treasures. At last, early one morning, when it was filled to overflowing, they returned to the rock castle and dragged the heavy bag up onto the rock where the Queen lay basking in the colours of the dawn.

The Sea Queen thanked them, then taking a handful of the beautiful shells out of the great netted bag, she tossed them far out into the waves that were rolling towards the shore. The waves took the shells and laughingly tumbled them along. Over and over they rolled them and tumbled them, until they were washed right up onto the golden beach. And there the waves left them, lying on the sand, pink and white and patterned bright, glistening in the morning sunlight.

Later that day, when Sandy the gnome was making his way along the beach, collecting sea-foam for his pancake dinner, he saw the shell treasures lying in the sand. 'Oh thank-you, thank-you, sparkling sea, for bringing these beautiful treasures to me', he cried as he picked them up, slowly looking at them inside and out, admiring their colours and their beauty. He then filled his pockets with them and returned to his sand-cave home. How excited he was to spread them out on his table and around his bed, his heart dancing with joy that his wish for beautiful treasures had come true.

Early the next morning, the Sea Queen tossed another handful of shells from her great netted bag into the waves. The waves took them and rolled and tumbled them along, until they were washed up high on the golden beach. And there the waves left them for Sandy to find, pink and white and patterned bright, glistening in the morning sunlight.

And from that day to this, early each morning, the Sea Queen tosses her gift to the little gnome who lives on her seashore and cares for her sea creatures. Old Sandy still collects some of the shell treasures for his sand-cave home, but he also likes to leave some for the children to find and take back to their homes, to spread out on the shelves in their rooms.

So if you go walking along a beach one day you may find a little shell, a gift from the Sea Queen herself, and you will know that Sandy the beach-gnome has left it there just for you, pink and white and patterned bright, glistening in the morning sunlight.

'Story bones' – The House that Had Enough!

New York: story idea for a seven-year-old child who was always uncoop-
erative in so many ways – if you asked him to turn on the tap he would
turn it off tighter, if you asked him to open the window he would try to
lock it instead!

A refreshingly funny story about a house that had had enough! –
when the wind blew the windows would open, letting in the cold
air – on a hot day the windows would stay tightly shut, keeping the
house too hot. When someone wanted to come in, the door would
stay closed, etc. No parts of the house worked together or helped
each other.

One day it began to rain – it rained and rained and rained – instead
of the doors and windows closing to keep out the rain, the doors
and windows opened and the water came inside, then the doors and
windows closed again. The house was full of water.

A helper (little mouse, little elf?) comes along and tickles (or tricks)
the windows and doors into doing the opposite. Everything in the
house starts working again – the rain stops, the water drains out of
the house, the sun shines, and the house is happy.

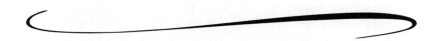

Endnotes

1   Van der Post, L. (1972), *A Story is Like the Wind*, p. 2, Penguin, New York.
2   Livo, N. & Rietz, S. (1986), *Storytelling: Process and Practice*, p. 5, L. U., Colorado.
3   Okri, Ben (1996), *Birds of Heaven*, p. 34, Phoenix: London.
4   Ken DiBenedette (2005), 'Metaphor at the Threshold', http://moonchalice.com
5   Antoine de Saint-Exupéry (1975), *The Little Prince*, p. 68, Scholastic Publications.
6   http://www.facebook.com/pages/Anandamayi-Ma/132031016894797
7   Kahlil Gibran (1972), *The Prophet*, William Heinemann.
8   Matthew 12:33.
9   Most 3- to 4-year-olds and some 5- to 7-year-olds. There is no precise way to determine the right age for a story, and some sensitive or more imaginative older children will still be fully absorbed by stories originally intended for younger children.
10 From *Healing Stories for Challenging Behaviour*, p. 6: There was once a young doctor who attended one of my storytelling courses, and in the introductory session, when it was his turn to say why he had enrolled, he told the group that for six years he had been at university studying medicine. As a consequence of this, in his words, his mind felt like a 'dried-up prune'. He was hoping that storytelling would help his mind become a 'juicy plum' again, as he remembered it had been in his childhood years. Over the next few weeks, starting with a simple story of the life of a carrot (with carrot seeds and a real carrot as story props) he progressed to telling and writing imaginative tales. This same doctor now has a reputation for being wonderful with children. He keeps a story-bag in his surgery and to help relax his little patients he pulls out a story prop (a paper frog, a little doll, a shiny pebble …) and tells a story about it while preparing the child for their check-up or injection.
11 Susan Perrow (2009), *Storytelling in African Teacher Training*, p. 150, Lambert Academic Publishing, Saarbrucken.
12 Nancy Mellon, *Storytelling with Children*, Hawthorn Press, ISBN: 978-1-903458-08-2.

Appendix 1

List of stories

Stories by Susan Perrow (not previously published)

A Doll called 'Rainbow'
A Doll from Heaven
A Lyrebird with a Cockatoo Voice
Baba Simba
Baby Hippo's New Teeth
Canoe Girl
Daisy White
Forest Boy and the Red Shoes
Grandfather's Cloak of Light
Heavenly Magic
King Flower
Little Gold Horse
Little Roo
Little Siafu and her Shiny Stone Drum
Panya the Rat
Saturdays
The Ants and the Storm
The Barnacle-Covered Fish
The Boat and the Dolphin
The Boy and the Pearly White Shell
The Bunny Clowns
The Digger that Always Says 'No'!
The Elephant's Trunk
The Frangipani Gift
The Golden Dolphin
The Golden Pipe
The Hare, the Parrot and the Bear
The Keeper of the Lake
The Leaking Roof
The Light of the Future
The Little Drummer Boy
The Little Pigs and the Hyena
The Not-So-Perfect House
The Ocean Playground

The Oriole and the Cherry Tree
The Party in the Jungle
The Princess and the Mirror
The Rainbow Horses
The Rainbow Dove
The Rhythm Sticks
The Rose and the Thorn
The Rosella and the Strawberry Patch
The Sailor Boy
The Scratchy Spiky Porcupine
The Shadow Giant
The Shouting Clock
The Shy Robot
The Singing Snake and the Dancing Bear
The Sparkling River
The Star Child's Journey
The Stick that Sings
The Tortoise and the Market Bus
The White Birds and the Rain
The Winged Horse
Twiga in the Mist
Wombat Helps to Build a Dam

Stories transcribed/rewritten by Susan Perrow:

Ariadne's Thread
Good Night, Sleep Well and Bless You
Hot Hippo
Kipury: An African Midwinter Story
The Bowing Tree
The Butterfly
The Children and the Butterfly
The Farmer and the Magic Stick
The King and his Three Sons
The Magic Cooking Pot
The Peddler and his Caps
The Story Bag
The Three Pots

Stories rewritten by others:

The Three Butterflies – rewritten from a traditional tale by Ellon Gold

Stories written by others:

A Family of Snails – Matthew Barton (England)

A Friend on the Farm – Edna Sophi Amunga (Kenya)
Big Things When You are Little – Natasha Hund (Australia)
Buddy Cuddle – Alfira Fisher (Australia)
Bully Bear – Aimee Chua (Philippines)
Clever Chameleon – Silviah Njagi (Kenya)
Juniper the Rabbit – Didi A. Devapriya (Romania)
Kuky the Kookaburra – Anatelyah Harari (Australia)
Little Elephant Does Not Want to Walk – Erika Katacic Kozic (Croatia)
Little Lead Pencil – Melanie Turner (Australia)
Little Wolf – Kim Davie (Australia)
Rainbow Colours – Janine Hutton (Australia)
Silvester the Snail – Alfira Fisher (Australia)
The Bees – Silviah Njagi (Kenya)
The Caterpillar – Marama Warren (Australia)
The Gnomes and the Golden Crowns – Silviah Njagi (Kenya)
The Gum Tree – Natalie (Australia)
The Lonely Robin – Stephen Sharpe (Scotland)
The Red Berries and the Handy Squirrel – Laura Hurtado-Roberts (New Zealand)
The Shining Star – Rosalind Veness (Australia)
The Thank-you Princess – Dawn Tranter (Australia)
The Three Ponies – Sue Hurst (New Zealand)
The Wandering Gnome with the Kind Hands – Dawn Tranter (Australia)
The Wombat Family – Kristen Palazzo (US/Singapore)
Winnie the Fussy Eater – Shan Ang (on behalf of Jumi, Shan and Ivory – Singapore)
Yogi and the Cobra Snake – Edi Ryagard (South Africa/UK)

Published by Immortal Books in *Gifts from the Sea* (1996, 2005)

A Gift of Shells
The Song of the Seashell

Published by Immortal Books in *The Knocking Door Tree* Forest Collection (2004)

Juju Finds a Friend
Mindy at the Country Fair

Published by Immortal Books in *Garden of Light* (2002)

Little Brown Bulb

Appendix 2

About the authors

Susan Perrow M.Ed.(Hons)

Susan Perrow is a 'story doctor'. She writes, collects and documents stories that offer a therapeutic journey for the storyteller and listener – a positive, imaginative way of healing difficult situations.

Susan has an extensive background in teaching, teacher training, storytelling and course facilitating. She was the founder and director for twelve years of Periwinkle Children's Centre in Byron Bay, Australia. In 2000 she developed a 150-hour unit on Storytelling for Southern Cross University and in 2001 she completed her Masters Research on Storytelling in a cross-cultural situation, post-apartheid South Africa. From 2001 to 2003, as the coordinator of a pilot program funded by the Australian Government under its "Developing Stronger Families Project", Susan developed courses and resources for Parent Support, specializing in storytelling and creative discipline. She now gives workshops and training seminars for teachers, parents and therapists around the world and online.

Her story work has led to the publication of three other books: *Healing Stories for Challenging Behaviour, An A-Z Collection of Behaviour Tales* and *Stories to Light the Night* all published by Hawthorn Press. These books have been translated into many languages, including Chinese, Korean, Japanese, Spanish, Portuguese, Slovenian, Serbian and Croatian.

Susan is a mother of three boys, and a grandmother to a growing number of children. Her home is in Lennox Head on the east coast of Australia.

Jennifer M. Gidley PhD

Jennifer M. Gidley, who wrote the Foreword, is a Research Fellow in the Global Cities Research Institute at RMIT University, Melbourne and is President of the World Futures Studies Federation. She is a psychologist, educator and researcher in the future studies field with a transdisciplinary understanding of global shifts in culture and consciousness. Her career includes working as a school and community psychologist, teaching principal, academic teacher and researcher over three decades and all educational levels and sectors.

Other books by the Susan Perrow

Stories to Light the Night

A grief and loss collection for children, families and communities

A unique, comprehensive collection of 94 imaginatively crafted stories for sharing at times of grieving, bereavement, separation or loss. The stories come from different contributors and from many different cultures worldwide. *'The stories in this book are deeply tender, consoling gifts for children and adults who are wounded by overwhelming loss. They matter. A lot.'* Alida Gersie Ph.D. Consultant to NHS Children's Hospital at Home Services, author and co-editor, *Storytelling for a Greener World* **192pp; 234 x 156mm; 978-1-912480-27-2; paperback**

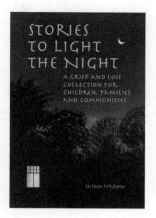

An A-Z Collection of Behaviour Tales

From Angry Ant to Zestless Zebra

This collection of 42 tales offers story medicine as a creative strategy for parenting, teaching and counselling. With charming illustrations the stories follow the alphabet from A to Z. *'Susan is a trailblazer for the movement for healing stories… you can adapt Susan's tales for your own situation or even create your own.'* Georgiana Keable, author of *The Natural Storyteller* **144pp; 234 x 156mm; 978-1-907359-86-6; pbk**

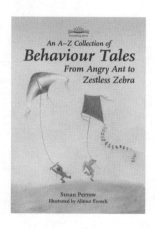

Healing Stories for Challenging Behaviour

Here are 80 stories for resolving common childhood issues, such as separation anxiety, bullying, sibling rivalry, nightmares and grieving. Accompanied with lively anecdotes, the book includes guidelines for creating new stories relevant to a reader's own circumstances. *'Susan Perrow's inspirational adventures with storytelling have grown into this inspirational book.'* Nancy Mellon, author of *Storytelling with Children* **320pp; 234 × 156mm; 978-1-903458-78-5; pbk**

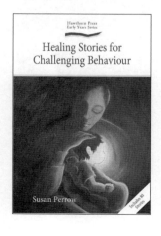

Other Books From Hawthorn Press

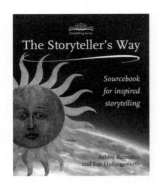

The Storyteller's Way

A Sourcebook for Inspired Storytelling

Sue Hollingsworth, Ashley Ramsden

To tell a story well you need a certain set of skills, and this book is an essential guide.

Use it to tell stories for entertainment, teaching, coaching, healing or making meaning. It contains a wealth of stories, exercises, questions, tips and insights to guide your storytelling path, offering time-tested and trusted ways to improve your skills, overcome blocks and become a confident and inspirational storyteller.

256pp; 228 × 186mm; 978-1-907359-19-4; pb

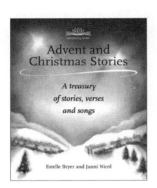

Advent and Christmas Stories

A treasury of stories, verses and songs

Estelle Bryer, Janni Nicol

From Advent and the Twelve Days of Christmas, to the flight into Egypt: Estelle Bryer and Janni Nicol tell their favourite Christmas stories. Their approach is simple yet profound and draws on their lifelong experience as Waldorf kindergarten educators, puppeteers, and as mothers. These stories will delight young children, and invite parents and teachers to become more confident storytellers.

128pp; 228 × 186mm; 978-1-907359-25-5; pb

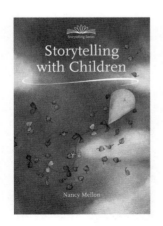

Storytelling with Children

Nancy Mellon

Telling stories awakens wonder and creates special occasions with children, whether it is bedtime, around the fire or on rainy days. Encouraging you to spin golden tales, Nancy Mellon provides methods, tips and resources to enable you to become a confident storyteller, by using the day's events and rhythms to make stories, transforming old stories and making up new ones, and bringing your personal and family stories to life.

192pp; 216 × 138mm; 978-1-907359-26-2; pb

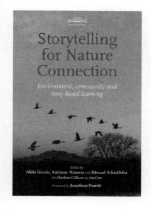

Storytelling for Nature Connection

Environment, community and story-based learning

Edited by Alida Gersie, Anthony Nanson and Edward Schieffelin

This handbook brings together the wisdom of cutting-edge storytellers in 21 chapters showing distinctive but complementary approaches to the art of telling stories for environmental education. It offers time-tested stories, creative activities and methods that environmental educators and storytellers can use to affect people's pro-environmental behaviour.

376pp; 234 x 159mm; 978-1-912480-59-3; pb

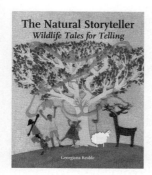

The Natural Storyteller

Wildlife Tales for Telling

Georgiana Keable

Here is a handbook for the natural storyteller: true stories of environmental heroines and heroes. Stories gleaned from the treasures of world traditions, but re-visioned for today's child. Includes story maps, brain-teasing riddles, story skeletons and adventures to make a tale your own; a vibrant invitation to embrace a world of stories all about nature, animals and plants – and our relationship with them.

272pp; 228 x 138mm; 978-1-907359-80-4; pb

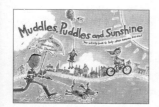

Muddles, Puddles and Sunshine

Your activity book to help when someone has died

Diana Crossley, Illustrated by Kate Sheppard

Beautifully illustrated, this book offers practical and sensitive support for bereaved children. Through a helpful series of activities and exercises it offers them a structure and an outlet for the many difficult feelings which inevitably follow when someone dies.

34pp; 297 × 210mm; 978-1-869890-58-2; pb

Ordering Books

If you have difficulties ordering Hawthorn Press books from a bookshop, you can order direct from our website **www.hawthornpress.com** or from our UK distributor:

BOOKSOURCE
50 Cambuslang Road
Glasgow
G32 8NB
Tel: (0845) 370 0063
Email: orders@booksource.net

Details of our overseas distributors can be found on our website.

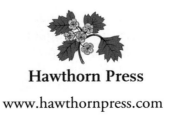

Hawthorn Press

www.hawthornpress.com